KT-468-792

Contents

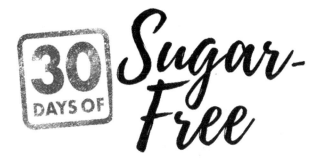

30 DAYS OF Sugar-Free

A whole month of delicious recipes to make going sugar-free a breeze

Catherine Kidd R.D.

First published in Great Britain in 2018 by Seven Dials
An imprint of Orion Publishing Group Ltd
Carmelite House, 50 Victoria Embankment, London, EC4Y 0DZ

An Hachette UK Company

1 3 5 7 9 10 8 6 4 2

Text © Catherine Kidd 2018

The right of Catherine Kidd to be identified as the author
of this work has been asserted in accordance with the
Copyright, Designs and Patents Act 1988.

A CIP catalogue record for this book is available
from the British Library.

Paperback ISBN: 9781841882857
Ebook ISBN: 9781841882864

Photography: Vincent Whiteman
Food stylist: Laurie Perry
Prop stylist: Rebecca Newport

Printed and bound by CPI Group (UK) Ltd, Croydon, CR0 4YY

Every effort has been made to ensure the information in this book is accurate.
The information in this book may not be applicable in each individual case so
it is advised that professional medical advice is obtained for specific health
matters and before changing any medication or dosage. Neither the publisher
nor author accepts any legal responsibility for any personal injury or other
damage or loss arising from the use of the information in this book. In addition,
if you are concerned about your diet or exercise regime and wish to change
them, you should consult a health practitioner first.

Every effort has been made to fulfil requirements with regard to reproducing
copyright material. The author and publisher will be glad to rectify any
omissions at the earliest opportunity.

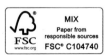

www.orionbooks.co.uk

Welcome to 30 Days of Sugar-Free!

Sugar-free is the ultimate trend at the moment – there are so many celebrities who have produced 'low-sugar' or 'sugar-free' books and there is a plethora of information available on the internet. I am a dietitian by trade, with a masters degree in nutrition, and I work for the NHS and in my own private practice; it seems that on a daily basis now I am asked by patients about what sugar actually is and how they can avoid it. They ask questions about processed sugar vs unrefined or 'natural' sugar, and they get confused over whether they should be avoiding fruit and certain vegetables because of something they have read. It seems that sometimes the information available about sugar is confusing or even wrong.

I believe that going sugar-free can be a really healthy option, and as a dietitian I wanted to offer advice and recipes that people could trust. The inspiration for this book comes from not only my patients, but also from a close friend who proudly told me she had cut out carbohydrates. She was, in fact, eating a packet of sweets whilst she told me. This made me realise that, in a world with vast quantities of nutritional information available at our fingertips, lots of good-quality information is getting lost among the 'fake news'. I thought this friend, as well as many others, could benefit from easy-to-understand and scientifically accurate information, to help them to reduce their unhealthy food consumption and avoid falling into the trap of following faddy internet diets. This book is not saying 'never eat sugar again' or 'sugar is the devil', but instead I hope it will help you to find a happy medium by reducing your sugar intake and enabling you to enjoy healthy meals balanced with carbohydrate, protein and fruits and vegetables.

Embarking on a new way of eating can be daunting – and sometimes expensive. What I have aimed to do with this book is provide a month's worth of recipes that will ensure that you get a varied, cost-effective diet with little waste at the end of each week, and to guide you to follow a new, balanced diet that is low in sugar.

WHAT IS SUGAR?

Firstly, let's clarify exactly what sugar is. Sugar is a molecule that is a combination of carbon, hydrogen and oxygen (which, incidentally, is what most of our body is made from!). There are lots of different types of sugar, so don't fall into the trap of thinking that sugar is just the white stuff that you put into cakes and biscuits. However, because there are so many different forms, you may not always be able to identify it on the ingredients list on a food packet. If you are trying to cut out sugar from your diet, here's a quick run-down of what you are looking for on those labels:

- A monosaccharide (*mono*- means one, *saccharide* means sugar) is a single sugar. There are three of these: glucose, galactose and fructose. Glucose and fructose are found in fruits, vegetables and honey, whilst galactose is generally found in lactose (see below).
- A disaccharide (*di*- means two) means two sugars attached

together. There are three of these: sucrose, maltose and lactose. The main sources of these are table sugar, malted sugar products and dairy.
- A polysaccharide (*poly*- means many) is when many sugars are attached together. An example of a polysaccharide is starch, more often called carbohydrate.

WHY PEOPLE CUT OUT SUGAR

There are many good reasons why cutting out sugar is a good idea for your health. Here are some of the main ones:

1 To lose weight
Eating lots of sugary foods can make you gain weight, as of course they are high in calories but also they often don't make you feel full so you will eat more than you need to. Fizzy drinks and sugary snacks take a lot of the blame for this, which we will talk more about later. Being overweight or obese has been linked with an increased risk of lots of diseases, such as arthritis and some cancers (including breast cancer). Keeping at a healthy weight can help protect your long-term health, and cutting back on sugar can be a big part of this.

2 Promote good dental health
Any dentist will tell you that sugar is bad for your teeth. This is because sugar feeds the bacteria in your mouth, enabling them to produce acid, which then causes your teeth to decay. Looking after your teeth by having a low-sugar diet can make a huge difference to your dental health, preventing lots of pain as well as costly dental bills.

3 To help **control certain diseases**
There are many diseases that can be prevented or treated by reducing sugar, such as heart disease and diabetes. On the other hand, there are also many diseases that have been falsely linked to sugar intake; hopefully this book will help dispel some of the myths for you so you know exactly what the benefits of cutting out sugar are.

Whatever your motivations for going 'sugar-free', there are two pros that are both universal and universally appealing.

It's easy

Preparing dishes that avoid sugar takes no longer than preparing food that is full of it. Once you understand which foods contain sugar and which don't, and how to read a food label for sugar-containing ingredients, you'll be able to whip up a healthy dinner in no time. This book is designed with busy people in mind – I'm always rushing around and in a hurry and I'm sure you are too! – so the weekday breakfasts should take no longer than ten minutes to prepare. The lunches and dinners often tie together, so that one ingredient can be used across the two meals to save you valuable time, either on the same day or across a couple of days in one week.

Cooking in bulk can really help, too – if there's a particular recipe you like, double the quantities and freeze half of it – some recipes here serve more than four and are marked with a batch-cooking symbol. If you are going to cook in bulk, you may want to invest in a few small freezerproof containers so you can freeze each portion individually to avoid wastage. Remember, though, you should not refreeze previously frozen food once thawed, for safety reasons.

It's delicious

Once you're away from sugar, there's a world of flavour to explore. Patients and friends of mine have been amazed that when they stop eating sugar, they start really tasting all of the wonderful flavours and spices in their food. Sweetness can be really overpowering and it is exciting to discover new foods and tastes. I love eating food from a variety of different cultures, as you will see in this book, which is full of inspiration from India to Lebanon and Mexico. The more flavours you discover, the more creative you can be in finding a different, healthier way to flavour your food.

What does going 'sugar-free' actually mean?

DISCLAIMER! I should say right now that sugar is found in varying amounts in almost all foods, so it is therefore impossible to completely cut out sugar from the diet. So in this book, when I say 'sugar-free' I mean a diet that ensures you're not adding *extra* sugar to your food that isn't naturally found in fruits or vegetables already – as well as ensuring that you don't consume too many of these naturally occurring sugars either.

Some foods are naturally high in sugar, such as honey, molasses and plant syrups (pomegranate molasses, agave, maple, date, corn and brown rice syrup). While these are often thought of as 'healthier alternatives' to sugar, in reality they are exactly the same chemical – just because they come from a natural source and are not processed to the same extent, doesn't make them any better. Your body will still use them in exactly the same way! My recipes don't use any of these sugar alternatives, which makes this book very different from lots of other low-sugar books.

The main foods used within my recipes that contain natural sugars are fruit and vegetables, milk and starchy carbohydrates. These are foods that many diets have villanised, but let's take a look at why it's important to keep them in.

- Fruit and vegetables contain a sugar called fructose. However, fruit and vegetables also have lots of other beneficial nutrients, including vitamins, minerals and fibre. Furthermore, the sugar contained in fruits and vegetables is held within the plant cell, so these are less damaging to your teeth (see below).
- Milk contains a sugar called lactose, but it also has lots of other beneficial health properties, such as being a good source of protein and calcium.
- Carbohydrates are important for your body to function, and in particular your brain. More on this later (see page 13)!

Essentially, this book is free of 'non-milk extrinsic sugars' – which is a long way of saying that it has no sugar in it that is not either naturally found in milk or held within a cell (such as in fruits and vegetables). However, fruit juices and smoothies are a slight exception to the rule. The juice of fruits and vegetables is the bit that contains all the sugar, so by squeezing out the juice from the plant cells (as in juice) or breaking apart those plant cells (as in smoothies), you are allowing that sugar to damage your teeth. Furthermore, the fibre that provides so much of the goodness of fruits and vegetables is completely removed in juice and cut up into smaller pieces in smoothies. Diabetes UK currently recommend that it is OK even if you are diabetic to have a maximum of a 150ml glass of juice per day or a small smoothie, but in my opinion the jury is still out on this.

As a result, this book does not contain any recipes for fruit juices or smoothies. Fruit and nut bars are similar, in that the fruit is blended, so the sugar is released from the plant cells and the fibre is broken up, which is why the snacks section does not contain any blended fruit bars.

Some foods contain extra hidden sugars – that's sugar that has been added in where you wouldn't expect it! For example, bread, yoghurt, cereal and shop-bought sauces. There are two ways to avoid this: either make as much home-prepared food as possible, so you know what's going into it, or learn to read labels really well. Most people opt for a bit of both. You'll learn more about reading labels on page 10.

The practicalities of going sugar-free

UNDERSTANDING HOW MUCH IS TOO MUCH

To reiterate, it is completely unrealistic to think you will never have sugar again. It is there in lots of food, and carbohydrates (which are essential for your body) are broken down by your body into sugar. Therefore, the UK government and NHS have published guidelines for the maximum amount of sugar you should consume in a day, to make sure that even if you have some, you don't have too much. 'Free sugar' (non-milk extrinsic sugar, see above) should not make up more than 5 per cent of your total energy (calories) per day. In real terms, this translates as:

11+ years	7–10 years old	4–7 years old	0–4 years
Max 30g sugar per day	Max 24g per day	Max 19g per day	No recommendations (yet!)
7 sugar cubes	6 sugar cubes	5 sugar cubes	

This does NOT mean that you can sit and suck that number of sugar cubes each day; it simply means that you can still eat foods that naturally contain some sugar (such as fruit as a snack, or milk on your cereal for breakfast), but not overdo it.

READING LABELS ON READY MEALS AND SNACKS

Everyone, now and again, wants to buy ready-prepared foods, such as snacks, sandwiches or even full meals. With the best will in the world preparing from scratch everything that you eat is hard work. Therefore, it is important that you learn to read food labels.

When you look at an ingredients list on packaging, the higher up on the list the ingredient is, the more there is of it in the food. For example, if sugar is near the top, you can guess that the food contains lots of sugar. But, as I've mentioned already, it isn't always listed as sugar, it might be called honey, crystalline sucrose, nectars (such as blossom), maple, high-fructose corn syrup, fruit juice concentrate/purées, glucose, agave syrups, dextrose, maltose, fructose, sucrose, molasses and treacle – to name just a few.

Food products often have 'traffic light' labels on the front of the packet. Calories, fat, salt and sugar are highlighted in green, amber or red, to indicate how much of each are contained within the food, giving you an overall picture of how healthy (or unhealthy) the food is for you. So if you're looking at a food label for the sugar level, you can go straight to the traffic light label. This is what each of the colours mean with regards to sugar:

Green – OK to eat	Amber – watch out	Red – eat in moderation
<5g sugar per 100g of food	5–22.5g sugar per 100g of food	>22.5g sugar per 100g of food

As an aside, bear in mind that even if the sugar box is green, indicating the food is not too high in sugar, if all the other boxes are red or amber, that food is not going to be the healthiest option.

COST

This book is going to encourage you to make various things from scratch, and while this might seem more expensive in the short term as you stock up your cupboards, in the long run it should work out cheaper (and, of course, healthier!) than buying ready meals. The shopping list at the beginning of each week should also help you to keep costs down, as each recipe is carefully written to make sure you reduce waste and use everything on your list.

Let's not forget that sugary food is getting more expensive, which is another good reason to cut back! At the time of writing, the UK government has just introduced a 'sugar tax' – that is a special tax of 24p per litre on drinks containing more than 8g of added sugar per 100ml, and 18p per litre for drinks containing 5–8g sugar per 100ml. What this means for us as consumers is that sugary drinks will become more expensive, an initiative the government hopes will make people think twice before buying the drink (and, in turn, help reduce their reliance on some NHS services, because of the link between too much sugar and various chronic diseases).

CONTROLLING SUGARY CRAVINGS

In early human evolution our taste buds helped us to test whether foods were poisonous, because these often taste bitter, whilst food with plenty of easily accessible energy – or sugar – for us to harness tastes sweet. It is for this latter reason that – most of us at least – like sweet food so much. When food was scarce, the fact that we liked sugary foods best and could digest them so easily wasn't a problem for our health, but now sweet food is so readily available it is a problem, because, as you already know, lots of high-sugar foods can cause weight gain and they don't fill us up as well as other foods (such as high-carbohydrate or high-protein foods). Furthermore, being repeatedly exposed to high-sugar foods can make you crave them more. Both our past history and our present environment are therefore making it pretty tough for us to put that doughnut down.

The good news is that you can adapt your taste preferences over time. The lifecycle of a tastebud is, incidentally, about thirty days long, so if you reduce your sugar intake for one month using this book, by day thirty-one you should be used to this less sweet diet and come to crave the foods you're eating instead. Interestingly, patients of mine who have reduced their sugar intake have over time started to find foods sweet that they previously didn't, such as fruits, vegetables and unflavoured natural yoghurt. So if right now you're worried that you'll never be able to follow a sugar-free diet because of your cravings, worry not! The more you reduce your sugar intake, the more your cravings will ease over time.

How to keep
'sugar-free' healthy

Cutting down your 'free sugar' intake isn't the silver bullet to having a healthy diet – there are a few other things you need to think about, too. It is important to have balance; this is really well explained by the Eatwell Guide, which is a pie chart of different food groups, showing how much of each you should be eating for a healthy diet. You can find this pie chart on www.gov.uk or by googling 'Eatwell Guide'.

STARCHY CARBOHYDRATES

Approximately a third of your diet should be made up from carbohydrates. Carbohydrates are a crucial part of a balanced diet; they are an essential source of energy and nutrients, such as iron, fibre and B vitamins. Each meal should be based upon a carbohydrate food such as:
- Rice
- Starchy vegetables (such as potatoes or sweet potatoes)
- Pasta
- Oats
- Bread
- Grains (such as quinoa, buckwheat or couscous)
- Breakfast cereals – some are very high in sugar, so check the label!

A portion of carbohydrates should be roughly the size of your fist when cooked.

Not all carbohydrates are equal, however, so it is important to eat carbohydrates of the right type and quality. A very simple way to work out if carbohydrates are of a good quality is to choose 'brown' varieties (such as brown rice, pasta and bread) over the 'white' varieties, as these contain more fibre.

Some people think carbohydrates make you gain weight; this view has been fuelled by the popularity of low-carb diets, such as Atkins, Dukan and South Beach. There has certainly been a rise in obesity in the Western world, which has coincided with an increase in carbohydrate consumption. However, it is likely that the type of carbohydrates (such as highly processed or refined and sugary foods) is actually the problem. Furthermore, healthy carbohydrates are often high in calcium, iron, fibre and B vitamins, so cutting out this food group from your diet could leave you deficient in these important elements. It is recommended that you eat 30g of fibre per day, and healthy carbohydrates will help you to reach this target. If you are considering a low-carbohydrate diet, or you are diagnosed with a health condition that affects blood sugar (such as diabetes or reactive hypoglycaemia) you should always seek the advice of a doctor or dietitian to ensure you are still getting the right amount of fibre, minerals and vitamins.

FRUITS AND VEGETABLES

Approximately a third of your diet should be made up from fruits and vegetables. Although these contain sugar, they are low in calories and very high in vitamins, minerals and fibre, so they are essential for the healthy functioning of your body.

It is important to eat at least five portions of fruit or vegetables each day. Sometimes the media will report mixed messages about having more than five – and while having more is great if you can do it, five is more realistic for some people. Fresh, tinned, frozen or dried all count towards your daily intake. Because each fruit or vegetable will have a slightly different balance of vitamins and minerals, it is important to eat a wide variety. An easy way to do this is to make sure your plate is colourful at each meal. Eat the rainbow!

One portion of a fruit or vegetable is:
· 80g of fresh/tinned/frozen fruits and vegetables
· Or 30g of dried fruits or vegetables. Because dried fruit has a higher concentration of sugar compared to fresh fruit, I have limited its use in this book. As an occasional treat, it's still OK, though!

Lots of people who want to follow a sugar-free diet avoid certain fruits and vegetables, but this is not advised in current healthy-eating guidelines because of the importance of a range of fruits and vegetables that you need in your diet to provide you with a good selection of vitamins and minerals. As I've already mentioned, the sugar in fruits and vegetables is held within plant cells, so it is not as damaging to your teeth as added sugars such as table sugar, honey or syrups.

As discussed on page 7, fruit juices and smoothies are an exception to the rule and should be consumed with more caution.

PROTEIN

Protein is essential for a healthy body because it features in all the cells of your body and is responsible for their growth and repair. Approximately a sixth of your diet should be made up of high-protein foods. Examples of high-protein foods include:

- Meat
- Fish
- Eggs
- Beans, lentils and chickpeas
- Nuts and seeds

In the Western world it is very unusual for people to eat too little protein – in fact, most people consume much more than they need. For the majority of people who do moderate exercise, all the recipes in this book will give you enough protein, but if you are an athlete you may want to talk to a dietitian who specialises in sports nutrition to check you are getting enough.

Proteins are made up from amino acids. All proteins are made up of a slightly different balance of amino acids, so it is important to include a range of protein foods in your diet, to ensure you do not lack any of the varieties. Furthermore, many high-protein foods contain extra nutrients – for example, meat contains zinc and beans contain fibre. Variety is essential, which is why I have tried to ensure that there is a broad range of different types of protein foods in this book.

It is currently recommended that you limit your consumption of red meat to a maximum of twice a week, due to the links between red meat and high cholesterol and cancer risk. It is also suggested that you include two portions of fish per week in your diet, one of which should be oily due to the beneficial effects of fish oils on your heart. The recipes in this book have been carefully collated to ensure that you can follow these extra healthy-eating guidelines.

This book uses quite a lot of eggs, as they are a good lean source of protein with lots of vitamins and minerals, too. The eggs used in this book are all large and free-range, unless otherwise stated. I recommend buying free-range eggs due to the environmental and animal welfare concerns regarding battery chicken farming.

DAIRY AND ALTERNATIVES

Approximately a sixth of your diet should be made up from dairy and/or alternatives. Adults need a good source of calcium in their diet once a day; children need it three times a day to support their growing bones.

Milk, yoghurt and cheese are great sources of calcium, which is crucial for keeping our bones strong. For adults, it is recommended you choose lower-fat options for dairy foods (such as 0% fat yoghurt and semi-skimmed or skimmed milk) to reduce the saturated fat content. However, for children who need more calories in a smaller volume of food, full-fat options are recommended. In this book, all the recipes that use milk and yoghurt have calorie counts calculated based on semi-skimmed milk and full-fat of all other dairy options, because personally that is what I like to eat and cook with – as that's what tastes the best! If you prefer to use different options, such as full-fat milk or 0% fat yoghurt, bear in mind that the calorie content of the recipes in this book will be different.

If you aren't keen on dairy or have an intolerance, there are plenty of good dairy alternatives available that are a great way to ensure you get your daily requirement of calcium. Examples include calcium-fortified plant milk (soya, rice, coconut, oat, hemp), soya or coconut yoghurts and soya cheese. 'Fortified' just means that a nutrient has been added to the food (in this case, calcium). Organic foods are not fortified, so, from a health perspective at least, it is better to buy non-organic dairy alternatives that have higher calcium levels.

Some dairy foods also have lots of hidden sugars, and yoghurts aimed at children or babies – fruit-flavoured fromage frais and flavoured milk – are often major culprits. Adding sugar can make foods more palatable, but getting children used to high-sugar foods from a young age could affect their food preferences throughout their life. Therefore, it is much better to choose Greek yoghurt with some fruit added.

FAT

Your diet should contain a small amount of fat. Fat is not only an important source of calories, but it is also essential for the healthy functioning of all the cells in our body – the outside of the cell (the membrane) contains fat and allows the cell to function properly. However, of course, too much fat can make you gain weight. Where carbohydrates and proteins are four calories per gram, fats are nine calories per gram (so more than double!). To help you maintain a healthy weight it is recommended that you limit your intake of fats as much as possible.

There are three types of fat: saturated, polyunsaturated and monounsaturated. As a rule of thumb, saturated fats are not good for our heart, while mono- and polyunsaturated fats are. This is because saturated fat increases your 'bad' cholesterol (fat going into your blood and around the body), while unsaturated fats can reduce your 'bad' cholesterol and/or increase your 'good' cholesterol (fat being transported out of your body). It is recommended that you focus on unsaturated ('good' or 'healthy' fats) and limit saturated ('bad' or 'unhealthy' fats) as much as possible.

In general, saturated fats are solid at room temperature, whilst poly- or monounsaturated fats are liquid at room temperature. In this book, unsaturated fats feature quite heavily – such as tahini in hummus, avocados, nuts and seeds, whilst saturated fats are limited.

Saturated fats	Monounsaturated fats	Polyunsaturated fats
Fatty cuts of meat and meat products, such as sausages and pies Butter, ghee and lard Chocolate Pastries, cakes and biscuits Full-fat dairy foods, such as milk, cream, cheese and ice cream Cheese, particularly hard cheese, such as Cheddar Palm and coconut oil	Vegetable oils, such as sunflower, hazelnut, olive, rapeseed, almond, peanut, corn, sesame and soya bean Avocados and olives Some nuts and nut butters, such as hazelnuts, macadamias, pecans, almonds, pistachios and cashews	Flaxseed oil (linseed oil is the same thing) Walnuts Rapeseed and soya bean oils Soya products Hemp-seed-based beverages Oily fish

You can limit foods high in saturated fat by buying lean cuts of meat and low-fat dairy, and by adding fewer fats, such as oils and spreads, to foods. If you do use fat in cooking, try to use unsaturated fats. For example, if you need to pan-fry a food, using olive oil rather than butter will be better for you.

There are two types of polyunsaturated fats: omega 3 and omega 6. Polyunsaturated fats not only have a beneficial effect on cholesterol, but long-chain omega 3 polyunsaturated fats also have an effect on the electrical impulses in your heart and therefore your heartbeat. Oily fish is the best source of omega 3 fats, which is why it is recommended to eat two portions of fish per week – one of which should be oily. Non-oily fish (such as white fish like sea bass, cod or haddock) are a good source of lean protein.

A lot of people struggle with high cholesterol, which can increase your risk of health issues such as heart attacks. Altering your diet to reduce your saturated fat intake and increasing your consumption of unsaturated fats can help. Lots of people who suffer from high cholesterol are also overweight, so for these people limiting the total amount of fat they are eating can be important, too, to help with weight loss. If high cholesterol is something that you struggle with, it is crucial that you seek professional advice.

Sugar: facts vs myths

So we know that there are health benefits associated with going sugar-free, but there are also plenty of myths about this way of eating. As a dietitian, I feel compelled to set the record straight here. So, what does the science really say?

What people say: Sugar is addictive

Myth or fact: It's complicated

I'm sure you have seen headlines in the media claiming that sugar is as addictive as illegal drugs. These headlines are highly sensationalised, but there is some science behind them. Lots of the studies that draw the above conclusion were carried out using animals such as mice and rats, so the results cannot necessarily be applied to humans; whilst we are all animals, our brains do not work in exactly the same way. However, there have been studies carried out with humans that show that sugar can cause cravings and then reward mechanisms in your brain that are similar to those caused by addictive drugs (like cocaine) – with some even concluding that sugar is more rewarding!

The complication is that we are designed to feel reward when we eat, because nutrition is an essential part of being human and staying alive in times of food shortage. We can't live without food, so some element of reward system in your brain is vital for life. Like I said earlier, the life cycle of a tastebud is about thirty days, so by reducing your sugar intake gradually you can wean yourself off a sugary diet. For this reason it has been suggested that quitting sugar is much easier than quitting other drugs and smoking.

What people say: Eating white refined carbs is as bad as eating the equivalent amount of sugar

Myth or fact: Myth

White carbs contain refined/processed grains (such as wheat and rice) where only the endosperm (inside of the grain) has been used and the husk (the outside of the grain) has been discarded. The husk is the part that contains lots of fibre, which slows down your absorption of the sugars in the endosperm. This means the sugars in white carbs are more easily accessed as they enter your digestive system as opposed to wholemeal/brown carbs, which is why people might be confused when it comes to saying white carbs are essentially just sugars.

However, you cannot compare eating a handful of sweets to eating a bowl of pasta, for a few reasons. Firstly, it is easier to take in more calories (energy) in a shorter space of time by eating sweets than it would be from eating white carbohydrates, which can lead to excess weight gain. Secondly, sugar is more damaging to your teeth than carbohydrates. Although carbohydrates are broken down into sugars, this doesn't all happen in your mouth in time to damage your teeth to the same extent. Thirdly, when you eat white carbohydrates, you normally combine them with some other food source that contains some protein, fat, fruits or vegetables, which makes it a more balanced option. And lastly, by law in the United Kingdom white flour has added iron, so suddenly your piece of bread or bowl of pasta gives you this essential mineral boost.

Having said that, brown carbohydrates are a healthier choice than white carbohydrates. They contain more fibre, which means they stay in your stomach longer and keep you full for longer. White carbohydrates have been blamed for much of the rise in obesity in the Western world. The recipes here contain some white carbohydrates, but mostly you will find brown, for this reason.

What people say: 'Diet' drinks are better for you than 'full-fat' ones

Myth or fact: It's complicated

If I had a patient who was drinking carbonated drinks on a regular basis, I would recommend switching to a 'diet' alternative immediately, in an effort to cut down on calories and sugar. However, long-term, this is not an advisable option for a number of reasons. Firstly, carbonated drinks are damaging to your teeth even if they contain sweeteners instead of sugar, as they are acidic. Secondly, there is an argument that having the carbonated drink, even if it is artificially sweetened, does not help break your taste for sugary drinks and, therefore, will not help you get into a long-term lower-sugar diet. At this point you may be thinking 'but sweeteners cause cancer!' but this is actually a myth – see below.

What people say: Eating sugar causes cancer

Myth or fact: Myth

There is a lot in the media about how sugar causes cancer. This is based on complicated science, which is often oversimplified to the point that the meaning is lost or completely changed. The truth is, cancer cells usually grow fast, and growing takes a lot of energy. The energy that cancer cells use comes in part from the food we eat – some of this energy comes from breaking down carbohydrates into sugar. So yes, cancer cells do use sugar to grow. However, they also use protein and fat – they don't just want sugar! The myth that cancer 'feeds' off sugar came about because if cancer cells need sugar, then surely cutting out sugar will stop the cancer cells growing? Actually, all cells in our bodies, and in particular our brain, use sugar (which they get from carbohydrates), so there is no way for our healthy cells to get the sugar and stop our cancer cells getting it.

Having said that, a diet low in sugar is often a healthier one, with a lower risk of being overweight. Although no diet can cure cancer, having a healthy diet and not being overweight is one way in which you reduce your risk of cancer.

What people say: Eating sugar causes diabetes

Myth or fact: It's complicated

There are two types of diabetes: 1 and 2. A hormone called insulin travels around your body in your blood, helping to control your blood sugar. It does this by acting like a key – opening the door of the cells in your body so they can let sugar in and use the sugar for energy. Type 1 diabetes refers to the inability of the pancreas to make insulin, while type 2 refers to the reduced ability of the body to respond to the insulin. They are very different diseases, and have different causes.

Type 1 is caused by your immune system destroying the cells in your pancreas that make insulin. Having a diet low in sugar will not affect your risk of developing type 1 diabetes. Type 2 is caused by many factors, including body weight, gender and age. Increasing evidence suggests that your risk of developing type 2 diabetes is also higher if your diet is high in sugar. For both types of diabetes, having a low-sugar diet can help you control your blood sugar. If you are diagnosed with diabetes, you should always speak to a doctor or dietitian for individual advice before making any changes to your diet.

What they say: All sugar is bad for your teeth

Myth or fact: Fact

Dental decay is the most prevalent chronic disease in adults and children in the UK. In fact, we spent £50.5 million on tooth extraction in the under 19s in 2015 and 2016. This is largely preventable, and having a healthy diet is a huge help.

All sugar is bad for your teeth, but some types are worse than others. The worst are 'sticky' sugars, such as toffees, that get stuck around your teeth, and sugary drinks and foods consumed outside normal mealtimes – this is because your saliva protects your teeth. The regularity to which your teeth are exposed to sugar is also important – regular exposure hugely increases your chance of tooth decay. Better types of sugars are those found naturally in fruits and vegetables, as they are held within cell walls and are less accessible to your teeth. As already discussed on page 7, fruit juices and smoothies, where the plant cell wall is broken down, are worse than whole fruits and vegetables.

The best way to improve your oral health is to brush your teeth regularly, cut down on sugary foods and drinks, and visit the dentist on a regular basis.

What they say: 'Natural' sugars, such as honey or maple syrup, are better for you than refined sugars

Myth or fact: Myth

The white stuff we call 'sugar' is actually sucrose, which is made up from an equal balance of glucose and fructose. Honey is made from more fructose than glucose, and agave syrup is entirely fructose.

Fructose and glucose differ in two ways: fructose is sweeter (so you don't need to use as much) and it causes a slower rise in blood sugar – it has a lower glycaemic index. Combined with the fact that sweeteners like honey and agave syrup are naturally occurring, they are often seen as healthier because they are 'unprocessed'. In truth, they are processed to get from their raw form in beehives and cactuses respectfully and into a plastic bottle in a supermarket, and your body will recognise and use the sugar in exactly the same way. Some people believe they contain more vitamins or minerals, which may be true, but in such small quantities that the difference in micronutrient content is not significant.

What they say: Artificial sweeteners are dangerous to your health

Myth or fact: Myth

Artificial sweeteners are found in so many things – some of which you would realise (such as diet drinks, sugar-free jam and cakes) to some you wouldn't realise (such as chewing gum and toothpaste). There are lots of different artificial sweeteners – and here are some examples:

- Sorbitol
- Sucralose
- Srevia
- Xylitol
- Saccharin
- Aspartame

There has been a huge amount of scaremongering around artificial sweeteners – particularly around them supposedly causing cancer. However, Cancer Research UK has recently published a statement saying: 'large studies looking at humans have now provided strong evidence that artificial sweeteners do not increase the risk of cancer.'[1]

So artificial sweeteners are not *dangerous* to health, but are they healthy? Possibly not. New evidence suggests that they could increase your appetite, therefore causing overeating, which leads to weight gain and obesity. Furthermore, eating them could cause you to continue to crave sweet foods. In my opinion it is better to get used to an added-sugar-free diet than rely on foods with sweeteners in them.

What they say: Dried fruit/nut bars and energy balls are good alternatives to sugary sweets

Fact or myth: It's complicated

There are many snack bars that are currently available that are marketed as 'healthy' – mainly because they only contain natural ingredients, generally being blended fruits, nuts and natural flavourings. On one hand, they are healthier options than

1 www.cancerresearchuk.org/about-cancer/causes-of-cancer/diet-and-cancer/food-controversies#food_controversies

a packet of crisps or a bar of chocolate, as they contain fibre, vitamins and minerals (from the dried fruit) and protein (from the nuts). However, there are two reasons why they might not be the healthy snack that you think they are. Firstly, it is very likely that they will be high in sugar. Admittedly, it is natural fruit sugar and so it is held within fruit cells, but it is still there. Dried fruit is much higher in sugar than fresh fruit, because when the water content is reduced you eat far more. Secondly, if they contain honey, maple or agave syrup or the like, then – as explained above – just because they don't explicitly contain white sugar it does not mean they are healthy.

How to use this book

RECIPE COUNT

The book contains 30 breakfasts, 30 lunches and 30 dinners, all organised in individual days over the course of four and a half weeks. If you would rather choose recipes by breakfast, lunch and dinner, you can use the Recipe Index on page 271.

SHOPPING LIST

At the beginning of each week there is a shopping list that gives all the easy-to-source ingredients that you will need to make the recipes for the next seven days. The aim is to use up all the food you buy at the beginning of the week, with minimal waste – which is good for the planet and your pocket! Each week starts on the Saturday to allow you to go to the shops at the beginning of the weekend (or on Friday night) so you are ready for the week ahead.

STORE CUPBOARD ESSENTIALS

The 'store cupboard essentials' section lists all the ingredients that are helpful to have in your cupboards at all times, and which you will use for many recipes throughout the book. In the first week you will need to invest in this list as well as the shopping list – but don't be put off! Anything you buy this week will save you time and money in the long run. And you might find you have lots of these ingredients in your cupboards already.

BATCH COOKING

To make this book as practical as possible, many of the lunches use ingredients that are leftover from dinner from the few days proceeding, or are deliberately made in bulk to be split over a few days. For instance, in Week 2 when you make sticky aubergines for dinner on Monday (page 106) you use up the leftovers in a wrap for lunch on Wednesday (page 116).

SERVING SIZE

Each of the main meals (breakfast, lunch and dinner) are designed to serve four people, unless stated otherwise. If you find that you eat a smaller portion or you are cooking for fewer people, you can always freeze the leftovers. Bulk cooking is a great way to make healthy eating easier and it can often be cheaper, too.

CALORIE COUNTS

I personally don't condone calorie counting, but I understand that it can be a useful tool for those who are trying to cut back or for those who need to make sure they're eating plenty. All of the recipes in this book have approximate calorie counts for one portion, but bear in mind that calories vary greatly depending on the size of the ingredients you're using and the brand of the product, so these are loose estimations.

SNACKS

As well as main meals, this book will also give you ten snack ideas. These are not included within the weekly shopping list, as you may want to have them at any time throughout the month! If you find that your body needs more calories than the recipes in this book give you, snacks are a good way to fuel you and are often particularly important if you are exercising.

EQUIPMENT

To make this book as practical as possible, you should not need to invest in any fancy kitchen equipment. Below is a suggested list of essential items:
· Vegetable peeler
· Set of saucepans
· Ovenproof dish
· Baking tray
· Mixing bowl
· Wooden spoon
· Tupperware boxes (if you want to take lunch into work or freeze extra portions)
And nice to have but not essential:
· Blender: this is useful for soups, but you don't need a fancy and expensive one. Equally, you can eat your soups 'chunky'

Store cupboard essentials

Oils, vinegars and sauces

- ☐ Olive oil
- ☐ Vegetable oil
- ☐ Cider vinegar
- ☐ Balsamic vinegar
- ☐ Sesame oil
- ☐ Worcestershire sauce
- ☐ Soy sauce
- ☐ Fish sauce

Carbohydrate staples

- ☐ Plain flour
- ☐ Rolled oats
- ☐ Quinoa
- ☐ New potatoes
- ☐ Dried breadcrumbs
- ☐ Wholewheat pasta
- ☐ Brown rice
- ☐ Risotto rice
- ☐ White rice
- ☐ Wholemeal sourdough bread, sliced (or other bread, if you prefer)

Herbs, spices and flavourings

- ☐ Salt
- ☐ Pepper
- ☐ Tomato purée
- ☐ English mustard
- ☐ Tamarind paste
- ☐ Harissa paste
- ☐ Tahini
- ☐ Sriracha
- ☐ Horseradish sauce
- ☐ Vegetable stock cubes/ stock pots
- ☐ Preserved lemons
- ☐ Chilli flakes
- ☐ Dried oregano
- ☐ Mixed dried herbs
- ☐ Ground cumin
- ☐ Grated nutmeg
- ☐ Fennel seeds
- ☐ Cardamom pods
- ☐ Ground cinnamon
- ☐ Dried thyme
- ☐ Paprika

- ☐ Dried fenugreek leaves
- ☐ Ground ginger
- ☐ Mustard seeds
- ☐ Cumin seeds
- ☐ Curry powder

For the freezer
- ☐ Peas
- ☐ Broad beans
- ☐ Ice cubes/ice-cube trays
- ☐ Sliced brown bread (I like sourdough!)

For the fridge
- ☐ Unsalted butter

Other
- ☐ Bicarbonate of soda
- ☐ Baking powder
- ☐ Chia seeds
- ☐ Vanilla extract
- ☐ Capers
- ☐ Cornichons

Equipment
- ☐ Muffin tin
- ☐ Loaf tin (approx. 450g)
- ☐ Steamer

Recipes: Week 1

N.B. Each meal serves four people
unless otherwise stated.

MENU

	Breakfast	Lunch	Dinner
Saturday	Banana and cardamom bread	Chicken gado-gado	'Turkey' turkey burgers
Sunday	Spanikopita (feta and spinach breakfast pastries)	Corn chowder soup	Pork and preserved lemon tagine with roasted kale
Monday	Strawberries, cream cheese and cocoa nibs on toast	Bruschetta with mozzarella	Artichoke, garlic and cream cheese pizzas
Tuesday	One-pan bacon and eggs	Nutty mango, avocado and quinoa salad	'Steak'wiches
Wednesday	Nutty granola	Broad bean, artichoke and feta salad	Herby salmon en croute

	Breakfast	**Lunch**	**Dinner**
Thursday	Plum and pistachio chia pudding	Smoked mackerel and new potato salad	Shepherd-less pie
Friday	Nutty 'carrot cake' porridge	Spiced carrot and lentil salad with halloumi and peanut dressing	Crispy fish finger sandwiches with homemade tartare sauce

SHOPPING LIST

Carbohydrate

☐ Large olive ciabatta (from the bakery section of most supermarkets)

☐ 4 wholemeal burger buns

☐ 4 brioche buns

☐ 1 baguette

☐ 1 pack (500g) ready-made puff pastry

☐ 3 large baking potatoes (e.g. Maris Piper)

☐ 250g packet of ready-cooked Puy lentils

☐ 500g new potatoes

Dairy products:

☐ 500g Greek yoghurt

☐ 300ml crème fraîche

☐ 2 x 200g feta cheese

☐ 250g cream cheese

☐ 1 x 150g ball mozzarella

☐ 225g block of halloumi

☐ 4 pints of milk

Meat, fish and meat alternatives

☐ 500g turkey mince

☐ 400g skirt/bavette steak

☐ 2 pork necks

☐ 4 skin-on salmon fillets

☐ 300g Quorn mince (found in the freezer section of supermarket)

☐ 2 skinless chicken breasts

☐ 200g pack smoked mackerel

☐ 200g rashers of unsmoked back bacon

☐ 400g cod goujons

☐ 13 eggs

Fruits/vegetables

☐ 200g kale

☐ 2 iceberg lettuces

☐ 6 lemons

☐ 1 bulb garlic

☐ 4 red onions

☐ 3 cucumbers

- [ ] 150g watercress
- [ ] 1 white onion
- [ ] 1 head of broccoli
- [ ] 5 carrots
- [ ] 500g spinach
- [ ] 1 bunch of spring onions
- [ ] 3 bananas
- [ ] 120g rocket
- [ ] 2 Braeburn apples
- [ ] 4 plums
- [ ] 230g strawberries
- [ ] 100g green beans
- [ ] 6 medium tomatoes
- [ ] 1 mango
- [ ] 1 avocado
- [ ] 300g chestnut mushrooms

Other – dried larder foods

- [ ] 280g jar of artichoke hearts
- [ ] 1 x 400g tin of red kidney beans
- [ ] 200g cocoa nibs

- [ ] 1 x 198g tin of sweetcorn
- [ ] 1 x 400g tin of black beans

Fresh herbs

- [ ] Mint
- [ ] Coriander
- [ ] Parsley
- [ ] Dill
- [ ] Basil
- [ ] Chives

Dried fruits and nuts

- [ ] 200g prunes
- [ ] 100g raw cashews
- [ ] 250g pistachios (200g to be used in Week 4)
- [ ] 600g sultanas (200g to be used in Weeks 3 and 4)
- [ ] 280g tub of peanut butter
- [ ] 100g Medjool dates
- [ ] 100g pecans

BREAKFAST

Banana and cardamom bread

This bread gets all its sweetness from the bananas and apples. The aroma of baking bananas and cardamom will make your kitchen smell great, too. This loaf keeps well in the freezer, so slice it and freeze each slice separately for an on-the-go breakfast or snack. It is delicious spread with a bit of cream cheese, too!

Makes about 12 slices (recommended serving size: 2 slices)
Under 250 calories

---

3 bananas
2 eggs, beaten
1 tsp vanilla extract
120g Greek yoghurt
2 cardamom pods

½ tsp bicarbonate of soda
½ tsp baking powder
200g plain flour
2 Braeburn apples, grated

---

1. Preheat the oven to 180°C/160°C fan/350°F/gas mark 4 and line or grease a medium-sized loaf tin (approx. 450g).

2. In a large mixing bowl, peel and mash the bananas. Then mix in the eggs, vanilla extract and yoghurt.

3. Next, grind the cardamom seeds. You can do this by bashing the two pods with a pestle and mortar, or if you don't have one, use a bowl and the end of a rolling pin or back of a spoon to crush them and release the seeds. Discard the hard husks so just the small black seeds from the middle of the pods are left. Grind the seeds until they form a powder, then add them to the wet dough mix with the bicarbonate of soda and baking powder.

4. Sift in the plain flour and stir thoroughly to combine.

5. At this stage, the mixture may look a bit dry, but don't add extra moisture, instead, add the grated apple. Stir thoroughly to combine and transfer to the prepared loaf tin.

6. Bake the bread in the centre of the oven for 45 minutes. At this point it should look golden brown on top. To check it is done, insert a skewer into the middle – if it comes out clean, it's cooked through.

LUNCH

Chicken gado-gado

This is a traditional Balinese salad usually made with tempeh and tofu, but here I've substituted chicken, which is equally delicious. I've also added quinoa to give you some slow-release carbohydrate to keep you going through the afternoon. There is peanut sauce leftover, but this will be used in two other recipes later in the week!

Under 450 calories

FOR THE SALAD
2 skinless chicken breasts, cut into thin strips
2 tbsp olive oil
Juice of 1 lemon
200g quinoa
100g green beans, trimmed
½ cucumber, cut into small chunks

FOR THE QUICK PEANUT SAUCE
280g peanut butter (crunchy or smooth, depending on your preference)
100ml soy sauce
Juice of 1 lemon
1 tsp ground ginger
1 garlic clove, minced
1 tsp chilli flakes
100ml water

1. Preheat the oven to 220°C/200°C fan/425°F/gas mark 7.

2. Start by baking the chicken breasts. Put the chicken into an ovenproof dish, drizzle with the olive oil and lemon juice and bake for 25 minutes.

3. Cook the quinoa according to the packet instructions.

4. Steam the green beans for about 5 minutes, then drain. Immediately pour cold water over them so they retain their lovely green colour.

5. Leave all the salad ingredients to cool.

6. Meanwhile, make the quick peanut sauce by mixing all the ingredients together in a small bowl.

7. To assemble the salad, mix the chicken strips, vegetables and quinoa together, and dress with 2 tablespoons of peanut sauce.

DINNER

'Turkey' turkey burgers

Turkey is traditionally eaten during the winter holidays (for example, Thanksgiving and Christmas), however, there is no reason why it should be limited to the festive season. Turkey is a lean meat, which means it is low in fat whilst still being high in protein, and here the meat is pepped up with some flavours inspired by the country of the same name. When cooking the burgers, use a non-stick frying pan so you don't need to use as much oil.

About 400 calories

FOR THE BURGERS
500g turkey mince
½ red onion, grated or chopped finely in a blender (keep the other half for Sunday dinner)
1 garlic clove, minced
1 egg
2 tsp dried oregano
Pinch of salt and pepper
1 tsp olive oil

FOR THE TZATZIKI
½ cucumber

180g Greek yoghurt
Small handful of mint
1 garlic clove, minced
Juice of ½ lemon
2 tsp olive oil
Pinch of salt and pepper

TO SERVE
4 wholemeal burger buns, sliced in half
½ iceberg lettuce, shredded

1. First, make the tzatziki. Start by grating the cucumber, then wrap it in kitchen towel and press down to drain some of the water. Put it in a mixing bowl with all the other tzatziki ingredients and mix well to combine.

2. Next, make the burgers. In a large bowl, mix together the turkey mince, onion, garlic, egg, oregano and salt and pepper. Combine well with your hands, then shape into 4 flat burger patties.

3. Heat the oil in a frying pan over a high heat, then cook the burgers for 5 minutes on each side. To check they are cooked through, cut into one of them – it should not be pink in the middle.

4. Toast the cut sides of the burger buns. To serve, place the tzatziki, shredded lettuce and burgers inside the buns.

Get ahead

The tagine for tomorrow's dinner is delicious when made the evening before, as this really allows the flavours to develop. So if you have time, get started tonight.

BREAKFAST

Spanikopita (feta and spinach breakfast pastries)

These delicious pastries will make you feel like you are in the Mediterranean! The herby filling goes so well with the flaky pastry – they are sure to look impressive but they are so easy to make. I use ready-made breadcrumbs and pastry for ease, but you can make your own if you wish.

Makes 8 pastries (2 per portion)
About 550 calories per portion

---

1 tsp olive oil
4 spring onions, thinly sliced
400g spinach
Small handful of dill, very finely chopped
200g feta cheese, crumbled or chopped into very small pieces
75g dried breadcrumbs

Black pepper, to taste
1 tsp grated nutmeg, or more, to taste
Flour, for dusting
½ x 500g packet of ready-made puff pastry
1 egg, beaten
Fennel seeds, for sprinkling (optional)

---

1. Preheat the oven to 200°C/180°C fan/400°F/gas mark 6 and prepare a baking tray lined with baking parchment.

2. Start making the filling. Heat the olive oil in a large pan over a medium heat. Add the spring onions and cook for 3–4 minutes until soft.

3. Add the spinach and allow to wilt. It should lose much of its moisture during this process, as the water evaporates.

4. Transfer the spinach to a mixing bowl and add the dill, feta, breadcrumbs, pepper and nutmeg.

5. On a floured surface, roll out the puff pastry into a large rectangle about 1mm thick, then cut into four equal rectangles roughly 10 x 15cm – you can always roll them out more if necessary.

6. Taking one pastry rectangle, arrange the filling down the middle, length-ways, to form a 'sausage'. Fold the edges up around the filling and use your fingers to press together, to seal. Cut off the ends of the pastry if the filling does not come quite to the end, then slice in half to make two shorter pastries. Repeat this step until you have made eight pastries.

7. Arrange the pastries on the baking tray, seam facing down. Slash the top of each pastry twice (this allows the moisture to escape), brush with the beaten egg and sprinkle with fennel seeds, if you like.

8. Bake for 25 minutes, or until golden brown. Serve either hot or cold.

Sunday

LUNCH

Corn chowder soup

Corn chowder is a really easy comfort food, but it differs from most in that it's low in fat. I prefer my chowder chunky, but you can blend it if you prefer.

Under 250 calories

1 tbsp olive oil
½ white onion, diced
½ tsp dried thyme
1 tbsp plain flour
800ml milk
1 baking potato, peeled and diced
3 spring onions, chopped

1 x 198g tin of sweetcorn, drained
Small bunch of parsley, chopped
Paprika, for sprinkling (optional)
Salt and pepper, to taste

1. Heat the olive oil in a pan over a medium heat. Add the onion and thyme, and cook until soft, about 5 minutes.

2. Add the flour and stir to coat the onion. Then add the milk a small amount at a time, stirring continuously so you don't end up with floury lumps.

3. Add the potato and bring to a simmer. Continue cooking for about 10 minutes, until the potato is tender.

4. Stir in the spring onions and sweetcorn.

5. Divide among four bowls and sprinkle with parsley, paprika (if using), salt and pepper to serve.

DINNER

Pork and preserved lemon tagine with roasted kale

Often pork is thought of as fatty, but actually the majority of the fat is on the outside rather than marbled through the meat. Therefore, when well trimmed pork can be a fairly lean option. The fruit and lemons here add a really unusual flavour. The further ahead you make this, the better, so if you can, make it one day ahead.

Under 350 calories

2 tbsp olive oil
½ red onion (leftover from Saturday's dinner), diced
2 pork necks, trimmed of all visible fat, then cut into chunks
Handful of dried fenugreek leaves

Small bunch of coriander, finely chopped
Small bunch of parsley, finely chopped
200g prunes, cut in half
200g kale
2 preserved lemons, each cut into eight
Salt and pepper, to taste

1. Heat the oil in a large casserole dish over a medium heat. Add the onion and fry until soft, about 5 minutes, then add the pork and cook for a further 5 minutes, until lightly browned on the outside. This will seal in the flavour of the meat.

2. Stir in the dried and fresh herbs and prunes.

3. Pour in enough boiling water to cover the ingredients and simmer on a low heat for about 2½ hours (if you don't have enough time for this, less time is OK but the pork won't have such a 'melt in your mouth' texture).

4. Preheat the oven to 180°C/160°C fan/350°F/gas mark 4. Wash and dry the kale thoroughly – it is important that there is not too much moisture on the kale or it will not get crispy. Tip the leaves into a clean tea towel and pat dry. Spread the kale evenly on a baking tray and bake in the oven for 10 minutes, until crispy.

5. Stir the preserved lemons into the tagine, add salt and pepper to taste and cook for a further 5 minutes to ensure everything is hot throughout before serving.

BREAKFAST

Strawberries, cream cheese and cocoa nibs on toast

Toast can be a healthy thing to have for breakfast, but so often it is covered in sweet toppings like honey and jam. This is an alternative with protein (from the cream cheese) as well as some fresh fruit.

Under 350 calories

4 slices of sourdough brown bread (from the freezer)	230g strawberries, hulled and thinly sliced
100g cream cheese (½ tub)	100g cocoa nibs

1. Toast the sourdough bread.

2. Spread each slice of toast with cream cheese then top with strawberry slices and cocoa nibs.

LUNCH

Bruschetta with mozzarella

Bruschetta is a traditional Italian open sandwich. It is full of flavour thanks to the garlic and basil, and the tomatoes give natural sweetness. Adding mozzarella gives you some protein in the meal, which is important for keeping you full for longer. If you don't have a toaster available at lunchtime, you can assemble this recipe on bread or make a sandwich at home to take to school or work. Just as delicious.

400 calories

6 medium tomatoes, cut into
    small pieces
½ small red onion, finely diced
2 garlic cloves, crushed
6 basil leaves, finely chopped,
    plus extra to serve

30ml balsamic vinegar
60ml olive oil
Salt and pepper, to taste
4 slices of sourdough brown
    bread (from the freezer)
1 x 150g ball mozzarella, sliced

1. Mix the tomatoes, red onion, garlic, basil, vinegar, olive oil and salt and pepper together and ideally allow to stand in the bowl for half an hour, so the flavours mix together.

2. Toast the sourdough.

3. Assemble the tomato mix on the toasts and lay over the mozzarella slices. Crack a little more black pepper over and tear over a few more basil leaves to serve.

DINNER

Artichoke, garlic and cream cheese 'pizzas'

These pizzas use ciabatta as their base, so they are incredibly quick to make. The garlicky cream cheese gives it a great flavour, but if you are short of time you can always buy a ready-made one (such as Boursin or Philadelphia). Serving this with a side salad means you get plenty of vegetables, too.

Under 400 calories

FOR THE PIZZA
Large olive ciabatta (from the bakery section of most supermarkets)
6 tbsp tomato purée
1 garlic clove
2 tsp mixed dried herbs
150g cream cheese
1 x 280g jar artichoke hearts, drained and cut into small pieces (save half for lunch on Wednesday)

½ iceberg lettuce, shredded

FOR THE DRESSING
1 tbsp olive oil
1 tsp balsamic vinegar
Juice of 1 lemon
Salt and pepper, to taste

1. Preheat the oven to 220°C/200°C fan/425°F/gas mark 7.

2. Cut the ciabatta in half horizontally, so it opens like a book, then in half across the middle again. You should have four pieces – one per person.

3. Spread the tomato purée thickly over the cut sides.

4. Put the garlic, herbs and cream cheese in a blender, and blend until smooth.

5. Sprinkle the artichoke hearts on top of the pizza and dollop over the cream cheese.

6. Bake for 10–15 minutes.

7. Meanwhile, prepare the salad. You can make the dressing by whisking all ingredients together, then pour it over the lettuce.

8. Serve the pizza with the side salad.

BREAKFAST

One-pan bacon and eggs

Bacon and eggs is a British breakfast classic, but here we've added some mushrooms for extra flavour and to give your breakfast a vegetable boost. And by cooking all the ingredients in one pan you save on washing-up, too.

Under 550 calories

2 tbsp milk

6 eggs

Pinch of salt and pepper

200g rashers of unsmoked back bacon, visible fat trimmed off then cut into small pieces

300g chestnut mushrooms, trimmed

4 slices of sourdough brown bread (from the freezer)

2 tsp unsalted butter, plus extra for spreading

1. Whisk together the milk, eggs and salt and pepper in a bowl then set aside.

2. In a pan over a low–medium heat, fry the bacon and mushrooms in the butter for about 8 minutes, until the bacon and mushrooms are slightly golden in colour.

3. Add the egg mixture and stir continuously for 3–4 minutes, until the eggs are scrambled.

4. Toast and butter the sourdough, then serve the eggs on top of the hot buttered toast.

LUNCH

Nutty mango, avocado and quinoa salad

This is my absolute go-to lunch. It is very easy to prepare, as well as colourful and delicious. The combination of beans and quinoa makes this dish high in protein, while the fruit and vegetables mean it is high in fibre, too.

Under 400 calories

200g quinoa
1 x 400g tin of black beans, rinsed and drained
1 mango, peeled, stoned and cut into cubes
1 avocado, peeled, stoned and cut into cubes

1 cucumber, cut into bite-sized pieces
Small bunch of mint, leaves torn
Small bunch of coriander, finely chopped
2 tbsp peanut dressing (from Saturday's lunch)

---

1. Cook the quinoa according to the packet instructions.

2. Assemble all the ingredients together, then pour over the peanut dressing and serve immediately.

Tuesday

DINNER

'Steak'wiches

These are a real family favourite; the harissa gives them a lovely heat without being too spicy, and the crunchy salad keeps it healthy, too. Pounding the beef first, as you do in this recipe, keeps it nice and tender.

Under 550 calories

3 tbsp olive oil
1 garlic clove, minced
90g pot harissa paste
400g skirt/bavette steak

1 red onion, thinly sliced
1 baguette
Large knob of unsalted butter
150g watercress

1. First, make the marinade. In a small bowl, combine 2 tablespoons of the olive oil, garlic and harissa.

2. Take the steak and, using a rolling pin, beat it to tenderise the meat. Then put it into a dish, pour over the marinade and leave for at least 30 minutes, but the longer the better.

3. Preheat the oven to 180°C/160°C fan/350°F/gas mark 4.

4. Heat a non-stick frying pan over a medium–high heat, and fry the onion in the remaining olive oil for about 5 minutes until soft, then set aside.

5. Meanwhile, put the baguette into the oven for 5 minutes until warm and slightly crispy.

6. Next fry the steak. To save on washing-up, you can use the same frying pan that you used for the onions. I find that 4–5 minutes, flipping the meat halfway through, is adequate for a medium steak (pink in the middle), but if you like it cooked more, keep it in the pan for a bit longer. When the steak is cooked, leave it to rest for a minute then slice it thinly.

7. Meanwhile, cut the baguette in half horizontally, spread the cut sides with butter and serve stuffed with the steak slices, the cooked onions and the watercress.

BREAKFAST

Nutty granola

This crunchy, nutty granola is a great way to start the day. It's easy to make and is a much healthier option than store-bought granola, which can have a large amount of sugar added to it.

About 400 calories

100g rolled oats	2 eggs
100g raw cashews	50g unsalted butter
1 tsp ground cinnamon	100g cocoa nibs
1 tsp grated nutmeg	

1. Preheat the oven to 150°C/130°C fan/300°F/gas mark 2 and line a baking tray with baking parchment.

2. In a mixing bowl, stir together the oats, cashews and spices.

3. Crack the eggs carefully and separate the yolks from the whites. Discard the yolks – or see tip below. Whisk the whites in a clean bowl until they form frothy peaks.

4. Melt the butter in a saucepan, then remove from the heat and pour the melted butter over the dry ingredients, stirring to combine and coat everything in the butter. Gently stir through the egg whites.

5. Spread the mixture over the baking tray and bake for about 30 minutes, until the granola is golden and crispy. When cool, stir through the cocoa nibs.

Tip: You can use the egg yolks in another recipe – especially frittatas or scrambled eggs as extra yolks – or freeze them for another day. Just lightly beat them with a pinch of salt (to stop them coagulating) and pop into a freezerproof sealed container where they will keep for up to one year.

LUNCH

Broad bean, artichoke and feta salad

This salad is really green and fresh-tasting; broad beans are actually legumes, so like other beans and pulses they are high in protein. The artichoke hearts give a distinctive and slightly smoky taste, whilst the feta really brings all the flavours together. It is one of the easiest and most delicious salads in this book and is a real lunch staple for me.

Under 300 calories

400g frozen broad beans
Artichoke hearts (leftover from Monday's dinner), roughly chopped
½ small red onion
1 x 200g feta cheese, crumbled
1 garlic clove, finely chopped
½ cucumber, cut into small pieces
Small bunch of mint, leaves torn into small pieces
2 tbsp olive oil
Juice of 1 lemon
Pinch of chilli flakes, or to taste

1. Boil the broad beans according to the packet instructions, then drain.

2. When dry, mix the broad beans with the artichoke hearts, onion, feta, garlic, cucumber and mint.

3. Combine the olive oil, lemon juice and chilli flakes, then pour over the salad to dress.

DINNER

Herby salmon en croute

**The creaminess of the salmon filling against the crispy pastry
makes for a lovely texture combination. I like to add lots of
pepper as it goes so well with the herby, lemony crème fraîche.
You can make puff pastry from scratch, but I think encouraging
people to cook family meals is all about making it easy, so if I
were you I would just buy it!**

About 500 calories

---

1 tsp olive oil

100g spinach

Zest and juice of 1 lemon

100ml crème fraîche

Pepper, to taste

Small bunch of dill, finely
  chopped

½ x 500g block ready-made
  puff pastry

4 skin-on salmon fillets

1 egg, lightly beaten

1 head of broccoli, cut into
  florets

---

1. Preheat the oven to 220°C/200°C fan/425°F/gas mark 7
   and line a baking tray with baking parchment.

2. In a saucepan, heat the oil on a medium heat and add the
   spinach. Cook the spinach down until wilted, about 4 minutes.

3. Remove the spinach from the pan and put it in a sieve. Using
   the back of a spoon, press the spinach to remove excess
   water, then return the squeezed leaves to the saucepan. This
   will stop your pastry going soggy.

4. Off the heat, add the lemon zest and juice, crème fraîche, pepper and dill to the pan. Stir to combine.

5. Divide the pastry into four even pieces, then roll the first piece very thinly into a oblong shape about twice the size of the salmon fillet, as you will be folding the pastry over to encase the salmon.

6. Place the salmon fillet in the centre of the pastry oblong, spoon a quarter of the creamy filling on top, then fold the other half of the pastry over the salmon and filling to encase it. Press down the sides of the pastry case to seal, make three slashes in the top (to allow steam to escape during cooking and keep the pastry crispy), then brush with a little beaten egg.

7. Repeat Step 6 until you have four little salmon parcels.

8. Place the parcels on the lined baking tray and bake for 20 minutes, until crisp and golden on the outside.

9. Whilst the salmon is baking, cook the broccoli florets in a pan of boiling water. After 3 minutes, drain.

10. Serve the salmon en croute with the broccoli on the side.

Get ahead

Tonight you will need to start preparing tomorrow's breakfast (steps 1 and 2). But don't worry, it is extremely quick and totally worth it for saving time in the morning

Thursday

BREAKFAST

Plum and pistachio chia pudding

This breakfast is a lovely combination of soft fruit and crunchy pistachios, and it's a beautiful colour, too! Chia seeds are a very good source of soluble fibre, which is essential for keeping your bowels regular, and it also has beneficial effects on cholesterol. You need to start preparing it the night before, but it's worth it as it saves you time in the morning.

356 calories

500ml milk
½ tsp vanilla extract
4 plums, stoned and chopped
   into small pieces

120g chia seeds
200g Greek yoghurt
50g pistachios, to serve

1. Blend together the milk, vanilla extract and plums and tip into a bowl.

2. Stir in the chia seeds. Refrigerate for 15 minutes then stir again, before covering and refrigerating overnight.

3. In the morning, remove the chia pudding from the fridge, divide among four smaller bowls, layer it with the Greek yoghurt and scatter over the pistachios to serve.

Thursday

LUNCH

Smoked mackerel and new potato salad

Smoked mackerel is a delicious way to enjoy fish – it is quite salty so I would recommend enjoying it in moderation, but as part of a healthy balanced diet it is fine. It is also quite a cheap fish option, and a good way to get in an extra portion of heart-healthy fats.

Under 350 calories

500g new potatoes, cut in half
100ml crème fraîche
1 tbsp horseradish sauce (you
   can add more or less, to
   taste)

200g smoked mackerel
   (peppered if you can find it!)
Small bunch of chives, snipped
1 iceberg lettuce, shredded
Small handful of dill

1. Boil the new potatoes until soft, about 10 minutes, then drain and tip into a large serving bowl.

2. Stir the crème fraîche and horseradish together in a small bowl.

3. Remove the mackerel from their skins and gently flake the flesh into the serving bowl with the potatoes. Add the chives, lettuce and dill, then stir in the crème fraîche mixture and serve.

DINNER

Shepherd-less pie

Quorn mince is a great alternative to red meat – it is high in protein but much lower in saturated fat. Often people don't even realise it is Quorn unless you tell them. This dish, with the sliced potatoes on top, is much prettier than the average Shepherd's pie and the top is lovely and crispy. Also, by leaving the skin on the potatoes you can add a bit more fibre and vitamin C.

Under 400 calories

3 tbsp olive oil
1 red onion, diced
2 carrots, diced
1 garlic clove, minced
300g Quorn mince (found in the freezer section)
1 x 400g red kidney beans, rinsed and drained
4 tbsp tomato purée
Pepper, to taste

1 vegetable stock cube, dissolved in 200ml boiling water
1 tsp chilli flakes (adjust to taste)
2 large baking potatoes, thinly sliced
Salt, to taste
320g frozen peas

1. Preheat the oven to 220°C/200°C fan/425°F/gas mark 7.

2. In a saucepan, heat half the olive oil. Add the red onion and carrots and cook until softened, about 5 minutes.

3. Add the garlic and cook for another 2 minutes, until aromatic.

4. Add the Quorn mince and cook for another few minutes, until thawed.

5. Tip in the red kidney beans, tomato purée and pepper. Stir to combine then add the vegetable stock and chilli flakes.

6. Transfer the 'mince' mixture into a baking dish.

7. In a saucepan, parboil the potatoes for about 5 minutes, until soft. Drain and allow to cool enough to handle.

8. Lay the potatoes on top of the dish, starting in the middle and spiralling out like a flower. Drizzle the top of the potatoes with the remaining olive oil and crack over some salt.

9. Bake in the oven for about 35 minutes, until the potatoes are golden brown and slightly crispy.

10. Meanwhile, cook the peas by boiling them for about 5 minutes. Drain and serve alongside the pie.

BREAKFAST

Nutty 'carrot cake' porridge

Breakfast is often the hardest meal to fit in extra fruit and vegetables, so here I've added grated carrot for a slightly unusual twist and to help you meet your five-a-day.

Under 350 calories

120g rolled oats	1 tsp ground cinnamon
700ml milk	1 tsp grated nutmeg
2 medium carrots, peeled and finely grated	100g sultanas
	100g pecans, roughly chopped

1. Heat all ingredients except the pecans together in a saucepan over a low heat, stirring continuously. After about 5 minutes, the oats should have absorbed all the moisture.

2. Divide among four bowls and top with the pecans.

LUNCH

Spiced carrot and lentil salad with halloumi and peanut dressing

This salad is naturally sweet from the dates and carrot, with some spice from the cumin and tanginess from the lemon. It is easy to make and is meant to be eaten warm. If, however, you are taking it to work or school, it is good cold, too.

Under 500 calories

225g block of halloumi, sliced
250g packet of ready-cooked
  Puy lentils
1 carrot, coarsely grated
1 bunch of coriander, roughly
  chopped
100g pitted Medjool dates,
  finely diced
2 tbsp peanut dressing (from
  Saturday's lunch)

1. Start by grilling the halloumi. Heat up a frying pan, and dry-fry each piece of halloumi until lightly browned on each side, about 3 minutes per side. Set aside on a plate with a piece of kitchen towel to soak off excess oil from the cheese.

2. Mix the lentils, carrot, coriander and dates together, then lay the halloumi on top and drizzle with the peanut dressing.

DINNER

Crispy fish finger sandwiches with homemade tartare sauce

Fish finger sandwiches are classic British comfort food. These are smartened up with delicious homemade tartare sauce and plenty of peppery rocket and cool cucumber to make sure you get some veggies in, too! The fish goujons are also grilled rather than fried, reducing the fat content because the fat drips off them whilst cooking. If you're short of time, buying the tartare sauce is fine too, just check the ingredients list for sugar.

Under 600 calories

½ white onion, very finely diced
1 tbsp capers, very finely diced
6 cornichons, very finely diced
¼ tbsp English mustard
100ml crème fraîche

Salt and pepper, to taste
400g cod goujons
4 brioche buns, sliced in half
120g rocket
½ cucumber, thinly sliced

1. To make the tartare sauce, use the back of a fork to mash the onion, capers, cornichons, mustard and crème fraîche together. Season to taste.

2. Grill the goujons according to the packet instructions.

3. Toast the brioche buns, and serve stuffed with the goujons, rocket, sliced cucumber and homemade tartare sauce.

Recipes: Week 2

N.B. Each meal serves four people
unless otherwise stated.

MENU

	Breakfast	Lunch	Dinner
Saturday	Blackberry and apple breakfast 'crumble'	Avgolemono soup	Chicken tamarind curry
Sunday	Rye bread with avocado, bacon and cherry tomatoes	Warm lentil and halloumi salad with a zingy preserved lemon dressing	Wholewheat pasta with roast pork meatballs and gremolata
Monday	Pomegranate and tahini chia pudding	Roast vegetable salad with kale and hazelnut pesto	Quinoa bowl with sticky aubergines, hummus and feta
Tuesday	Kale and Parmesan scrambled eggs	Bulgur wheat, feta and olive salad with hummus	Prawn and chorizo paella

	Breakfast	Lunch	Dinner
Wednesday	Caramelised banana and cocoa nib porridge	Aubergine, sweetcorn and avocado wraps	Salmon tacos
Thursday	Healthy beans on toast	Nutty kale and chorizo salad with sriracha	Sweet potato burgers with a melting goat's cheese centre
Friday	Raspberry, almond and mint chia pudding	Soft cheese and roasted cherry tomato tartine	Chicken, sweet potato and tarragon traybake

SHOPPING LIST

Carbohydrate

- [ ] 4 chapatis
- [ ] 8 hard-shell tacos
- [ ] 4 wholemeal burger buns
- [ ] 220g bulgar wheat
- [ ] 4 wholewheat tortilla wraps
- [ ] Sliced rye bread
- [ ] 1 x 250g packet of ready-cooked Puy lentils

Dairy products

- [ ] 450g feta cheese
- [ ] 2 small goat's cheese rounds
- [ ] 150g soft cheese with garlic
- [ ] 100g soured cream
- [ ] 250g Cheddar
- [ ] 250g Greek yoghurt
- [ ] 2 pints of milk
- [ ] 1 x 250g block of halloumi

Meat, fish and meat alternatives

- [ ] 3 skinless chicken breasts
- [ ] 400g good-quality pork mince
- [ ] 4 salmon fillets (approx. 500g)
- [ ] 400g frozen prawns
- [ ] 200g chorizo
- [ ] 8 chicken thighs, with skin on
- [ ] 1 litre good-quality chicken stock
- [ ] 8 rashers of unsmoked back bacon
- [ ] 12 eggs (this will give you some leftovers for next week!)

Fruits/vegetables

- [ ] 6 red onions
- [ ] 3 white onions
- [ ] 2 bulbs garlic
- [ ] 3 limes
- [ ] 300g rocket

- [ ] 9 lemons
- [ ] 4 aubergines
- [ ] 7 avocados
- [ ] 6 tomatoes
- [ ] 8 sweet potatoes
- [ ] 300g green beans
- [ ] 4 courgettes
- [ ] 3 peppers (red, orange, yellow or green – according to personal preference)
- [ ] 500g kale, large stems removed
- [ ] 500g cherry tomatoes
- [ ] 3 apples
- [ ] 400g frozen blackberries (fresh is fine – just normally more expensive)
- [ ] 200g pomegranate seeds
- [ ] 200g raspberries
- [ ] 4 bananas

Other – dried larder foods

- [ ] 2 x 400g tins of chickpeas
- [ ] 4 × 400g tins of chopped tomatoes
- [ ] 1 × 400g tin of coconut milk
- [ ] 1 x 350g can of green olives
- [ ] 1 x 330g tin of sweetcorn
- [ ] 1.5 litres hazelnut milk
- [ ] 2 x 400g tins of butter beans

Fresh herbs:

- [ ] Root ginger
- [ ] Coriander
- [ ] Parsley
- [ ] Tarragon
- [ ] Basil
- [ ] Mint

Dried fruits and nuts

- [ ] 100g hazelnuts (use 50g in week 4)
- [ ] 300g flaked almonds (use 50g in week 3)
- [ ] 100g sesame seeds
- [ ] 150g cocoa nibs

Saturday

BREAKFAST

Blackberry and apple breakfast 'crumble'

Crumble is normally a traditional Sunday lunch dessert recipe, but why not try it for breakfast? It contains lots of fruit for natural sweetness, and oats give you slow-release energy to keep you going through the day.

Under 450 calories

200g rolled oats
50g plain flour
¼ tsp ground cinnamon
Pinch of salt
100g unsalted butter, softened
3 apples, peeled and chopped
   into bite-sized chunks

400g frozen blackberries,
   thawed
50g flaked almonds, to
   decorate
250g Greek yoghurt, to serve

---

1. Preheat the oven to 180°C/160°C fan/350°F/gas mark 4.

2. Combine the oats, flour, cinnamon and salt in a bowl. Add the butter and rub it in with your fingers until the mixture looks like breadcrumbs.

3. Arrange all the fruit in the bottom of an ovenproof bowl, and sprinkle the crumble over the top. Use individual ramekins if you have them, but if not a larger ovenproof bowl will be fine (it just doesn't look quite as pretty!).

4. Bake for 25 minutes, until the crumble is slightly golden.

5. Place the almonds in a shallow frying pan over a medium heat. Stirring regularly, cook them for 3–5 minutes, until golden brown. Be very careful as they burn quickly.

6. To serve, dollop Greek yoghurt on top and sprinkle with the almonds.

LUNCH

Avgolemono soup

This traditional Greek soup is a real crowdpleaser and reminds me of being on holiday. It is also a great way to use any stock you make after roasting a whole chicken. If you don't have homemade, I recommend buying the best-quality chicken stock you can – definitely use fresh rather than stock cubes as it provides so much of the flavour of the soup.

Under 300 calories

100g white rice
2 tbsp olive oil
½ white onion, finely diced
1 litre good-quality chicken
 stock
1 skinless chicken breast, cut
 into very fine strips

2 eggs
Juice of ½ lemon
Salt and pepper, to taste
Handful of parsley, finely
 chopped, to serve

1. Cook the rice according to the packet instructions, then drain and set aside.

2. Next, in a saucepan large enough to hold all the soup, heat the olive oil and fry the onion for about 5 minutes, until soft, translucent and aromatic.

3. Add the chicken stock and bring to a simmer.

4. Add the chicken to the pan and cook through, about 8 minutes. Cutting the chicken breast as fine as possible means it cooks quicker.

5. In a mixing bowl, whisk the eggs together with the lemon juice. Whilst continuing to whisk with one hand, ladle 2 tablespoons of the hot broth into the eggs (1 ladle at a time).

6. Then whisk the egg mixture into the soup – this will serve as a thickener. Add salt and pepper to taste.

7. Divide among four bowls and serve immediately scattered with parsley.

Saturday

DINNER

Chicken tamarind curry

This easy curry is a firm favourite – the tamarind gives it an unusual little 'kick'. Using both chicken and chickpeas gives you a combination of animal and plant protein, and makes the dish cheaper, too, because you need less chicken! I serve chapatis instead of naan breads alongside, as naan is made with butter or ghee and therefore much higher in fat.

450 calories

1 tbsp olive oil
1 red onion, diced
1 garlic clove, minced
Thumb-sized piece of fresh
    ginger, grated
1 tsp chilli flakes
2 tsp fennel seeds
2 tsp mustard seeds
2 skinless chicken breasts, cut
    into strips
1 x 400g tin of chickpeas,
    rinsed and drained

1 × 400g tin of good-quality
    chopped tomatoes
1 × 400g tin of coconut milk
2 tbsp tamarind paste
100g rocket
Juice of 2 limes
4 chapatis
Small handful of coriander,
    chopped, to garnish
    (optional)

1. In a large saucepan, heat the olive oil and add the onion, garlic and ginger. Cook on a medium heat, stirring regularly, for about 5 minutes, until the garlic and onion are tender.

2. Add the chilli, fennel and mustard seeds and cook for a further 2 minutes, until aromatic.

3. Add the chicken strips and cook for a further 5 minutes, until the chicken is cooked through (it should be white throughout).

4. Add the chickpeas, chopped tomatoes, coconut milk and tamarind paste. Put the lid on the saucepan, and leave to simmer for about 20 minutes. If you have more time, you can cook it longer and slower, which really allows the flavours to develop.

5. When you are ready to serve, stir in the rocket and lime juice.

6. Warm the chapatis according to the packet instructions.

7. Serve the curry in a shallow bowl with a little coriander on top, if you like.

BREAKFAST

Rye bread with avocado, bacon and cherry tomatoes

Rye is an ancient grain, and is delicious in bread. Personally, I only like rye bread toasted, as it has a tougher consistency than other breads. Here, toasted and topped with creamy avocados, it is delicious. This recipe contains bacon – provided it is well trimmed of fat and grilled rather than fried it is OK to enjoy this in moderation.

Under 450 calories

8 rashers of unsmoked back
  bacon, with visible fat
  trimmed
250g cherry tomatoes
1 tbsp olive oil
1 tsp dried oregano

4 avocados, halved and stoned
Juice of ½ lemon
Pepper, to taste
4 slices of rye bread
Chilli flakes, to garnish

1. Preheat the oven to 180°C/160°C fan/350°F/gas mark 4.

2. Lay the bacon on a wire rack in a roasting tin so that the rashers don't overlap – the fat will drip off the bacon during cooking, which you can discard.

3. Place the cherry tomatoes in a separate tin. Drizzle over half of the olive oil and scatter over the oregano, then shake the tin so the tomatoes are well coated.

4. Roast the bacon and cherry tomatoes for 15 minutes each (longer if you like crispy bacon).

5. To prepare the avocado, scoop the flesh out of the skins and mash it in a bowl with the lemon juice, the remaining olive oil and pepper. You don't need to add salt, as the bacon is high in salt.

6. Toast the rye bread.

7. To serve, top the rye bread with the mashed avocado, bacon and tomatoes. Crack a bit of pepper on top and sprinkle with chilli flakes to serve.

Sunday

LUNCH

Warm lentil and halloumi salad with a zingy preserved lemon dressing

This salad can be eaten cold, but I think hot salads are delicious and add a bit of variety! The lentils and halloumi provide filling protein, whilst the courgette provides some fibre and the preserved lemon gives the whole dish some 'zing'.

Under 400 calories

1 tbsp olive oil
½ onion (use leftover from Saturday's lunch), finely diced
2 courgettes, thinly sliced
1 x 250g packet of ready-cooked Puy lentils
1 x 250g block of halloumi, thinly sliced

FOR THE DRESSING
Juice of ½ lemon (leftover from Saturday lunch)
1 preserved lemon, finely chopped
Small bunch of parsley, finely chopped
1 garlic clove, minced
2 tbsp olive oil

1. Start by making the dressing. Combine all ingredients together in a bowl and set aside.

2. Heat the olive oil over a medium heat and add the onion. Cook for about 3 minutes, until the onion is beginning to get aromatic and soften slightly. Add the courgettes and pan-fry for a remaining 8 minutes, until soft and golden brown on the outside. Add the lentils, stir to combine with the courgettes and onion and cook until they are warmed through. Set aside to keep warm under a tea towel or some tin foil.

3. Pan-fry the halloumi on each side, for about 2–3 minutes, until beginning to look golden brown.

4. Assemble the salad by dividing the lentils among four plates, then top with the halloumi and drizzle over the dressing. Serve immediately.

DINNER

Wholewheat pasta with roast pork meatballs and gremolata

Gremolata is an Italian garnish of raw, finely chopped garlic, parsley and lemon zest. It is really strong and adds a great, zesty flavour – it is one of my favourite additions to a meat or fish dish. Using wholewheat pasta here means that you get some extra fibre.

About 650 calories

FOR THE MEATBALLS
1 egg
2 tsp dried thyme
100g breadcrumbs
400g good-quality pork mince
1 tbsp olive oil

FOR THE GREMOLATA
1 garlic clove, chopped
Zest and juice of 2 lemons
Large bunch of parsley, finely
   chopped

300g dried wholewheat pasta

1. Start by making the meatballs. In a large bowl, whisk the egg then add the thyme, breadcrumbs and mince – breaking up the meat with a fork. Mix thoroughly to combine, then shape into small balls – you should have about 20 in total (five per person). Squash each meatball slightly – by having a flat bottom, they will be easier to cook.

2. Heat the oil in a shallow frying pan and fry each meatball for about 5 minutes per side, until browned on the outside and cooked through.

3. Cook the pasta according to the packet instructions.

4. Meanwhile, make the gremolata by combining all the ingredients and mixing well.

5. To serve, divide the pasta among four shallow bowls or plates, top with the pork meatballs and garnish with the gremolata.

Get ahead

It is a good idea to start making the base of the chia pudding now for breakfast tomorrow. This gives the chia seeds time overnight to expand and I think it adds to the flavour, too!

BREAKFAST

Pomegranate and tahini chia pudding

This breakfast is very quick to make, as the majority of it can be made the night before. You can even make a larger batch for a go-to breakfast as it will keep in the fridge for a few days. Chia seeds are a great source of soluble fibre, which is important for healthy bowels and can help with high cholesterol.

Under 400 calories

750ml hazelnut milk
270g chia seeds
1 tsp vanilla extract

1 heaped tbsp tahini
200g pomegranate seeds

1. Combine the hazelnut milk, chia seeds, vanilla extract and tahini in a jar or bowl and set in the fridge for 15 minutes, then remove and mix again. Cover the bowl or jar with a lid or cling film and return to the fridge overnight.

2. In the morning, remove the chia pudding from the fridge, divide among four bowls, then top each with the pomegranate seeds to serve.

Monday

LUNCH

Roast vegetable salad with kale and hazelnut pesto

This lunch is equally delicious hot or cold. If you don't want to make the pesto yourself you can buy it – look in the fresh pasta section of the supermarket. The roasted vegetables are deliciously sweet and full of antioxidants, and go well with the salty cheese.

About 450 calories

FOR THE ROASTED VEGETABLES
2 courgettes, cut into half-moon chunks
2 peppers (red, orange, yellow or green – according to personal preference), deseeded and sliced
2 red onions, cut into half moons
4 garlic cloves, crushed
3 sweet potatoes, peeled and cut into cubes
2 tbsp olive oil

Pinch of salt and pepper

FOR THE PESTO
150g kale, large stems removed
50g hazelnuts, toasted
2 garlic cloves, peeled
Zest and juice of 1 lemon
4 tbsp olive oil

TO SERVE
Small bunch of parsley, chopped
150g feta cheese, crumbled

1. Preheat the oven to 220°C/200°C fan/425°F/gas mark 7.

2. Put the courgettes, peppers, red onions, garlic and sweet
    potatoes in a baking dish. Drizzle over the olive oil and add
    a pinch of salt and pepper, then massage the ingredients
    with the oil until all are well coated. Bake in the oven for 30
    minutes.

3. To make the pesto, blitz together all the dry ingredients in
    a blender, scraping down the sides of the bowl part way
    through if necessary. Then add the lemon juice and olive
    oil a little at a time while the blender is running, until well
    combined.

4. Once cooked, divide the vegetables among four separate
    plates and drizzle with the pesto. Scatter over the parsley and
    feta to serve.

DINNER

Quinoa bowl with sticky aubergines, hummus and feta

Often aubergines are cooked in lots of oil, which makes them a very high-calorie food. However, they are equally delicious pan-fried and are a great meat alternative for this veggie dish.

Under 600 calories

FOR THE HUMMUS
1 x 400g tin of chickpeas,
    rinsed and drained
3 tbsp olive oil
Juice of 1 lemon
2 tsp tahini
1 tsp paprika
1 tsp ground cumin
3 tbsp water

200g quinoa

FOR THE STICKY
AUBERGINES
1 tbsp olive oil
4 aubergines, cut into cubes
2 heaped tsp harissa paste

TO SERVE
150g feta cheese, crumbled
Small bunch of coriander, finely
    chopped
100g sesame seeds

1. Start by making the hummus. Tip the chickpeas, olive oil, lemon juice, tahini, paprika and cumin into a blender and blitz together until completely smooth. Add the water, a small amount at a time, until you reach the desired consistency.

2. Cook the quinoa according to the packet instructions.

3. Meanwhile, in a large frying pan, heat the olive oil over a medium heat. Add the aubergines and stir to coat in the hot oil. Fry for about 10 minutes, until they begin to shrink, brown on all sides and go tender.

4. Add the harissa paste to the aubergines and stir to coat. Fry for a further 2 minutes.

5. To serve, pile the quinoa into separate bowls and top with half the aubergines, saving the rest for Wednesday's lunch. Dollop 1 tablespoon of hummus onto each portion (saving the rest for Tuesday's lunch). Serve scattered with feta, coriander and sesame seeds.

Tuesday

BREAKFAST

Kale and Cheddar scrambled eggs

Kale is a great source of folate and gives these scrambled eggs lots of flavour and texture. I would recommend ripping off and discarding any of the tougher stalks from the kale and chopping the leaves finely. If you have any leftover kale, roast it as a delicious snack.

350 calories

1 tbsp unsalted butter
2 large handfuls of kale, tough
  stalks discarded
4 eggs, beaten

100g grated Cheddar
4 slices of sourdough bread,
  toasted

1. In a pan over a low–medium heat, add the butter and sweat down the kale for about 5 minutes, until very soft.

2. Add the eggs and stir, slowly, until scrambled, about 4 minutes. Then add the grated cheese, stir to combine and remove from the heat.

3. Remove the eggs from the pan and pile on top of hot toast to serve.

LUNCH

Bulgur wheat, feta and olive salad with hummus

Bulgur wheat is a traditional Middle Eastern grain, made from the groats of several different wheat species. It is a good source of plant-based protein and is high in minerals such as iron. If you struggle to find bulgur wheat at the supermarket, you can always substitute it with couscous.

450 calories

220g bulgur wheat

100g rocket

1 x 350g tin of green olives, rinsed, drained and roughly chopped

150g feta cheese

8 tbsp hummus (from Monday's dinner)

1. Cook the bulgur wheat according to the packet instructions.

2. Mix the rocket and olives into the bulgar wheat.

3. Divide the grains among four plates, crumble over the feta cheese and serve with hummus on the side.

Get ahead

You will need to defrost prawns now ready for tonight's dinner. It is best to do this slowly, by taking them out of the freezer and putting them in the fridge. Make sure you put the bag in a dish, as some water may be released from the prawns during the thawing process. If you don't think you'll be able to do this during the day, you can do it the night before, leaving them in the fridge.

DINNER

Prawn and chorizo paella

This is a traditional Spanish recipe and one of my go-to easy suppers. Chorizo is high in salt and saturated (bad) fat, so it is best enjoyed in moderation. Luckily it tastes so strong you only need to use a tiny bit of it.

Under 500 calories

1 tsp olive oil
1 white onion, diced
2 garlic cloves, minced
200g chorizo (for dinner tonight and for lunch on Thursday)
300g risotto rice
1 x 400g tin of chopped tomatoes

2 vegetable stock cubes, dissolved in 900ml boiling water
400g frozen prawns, defrosted
Juice of 1 lemon
Pepper, to taste
Small handful of fresh parsley, chopped

1. In a large pan, heat the olive oil. Fry the onion, garlic and chorizo, until the onions and garlic are soft and the chorizo has started to release some of its juices. This will take about 5 minutes. Set half of this aside for Thursday's salad.

2. Add the risotto rice to the pan and stir to coat in the chorizo juices.

3. Stir in the chopped tomatoes, then pour in a small amount of the stock, about 50ml at a time, stirring slowly to allow the rice to absorb the moisture. When all the stock has been added (this will take about 15 minutes), add the prawns and cook for a further 5 minutes, until the prawns are cooked through. If you are using ready-cooked ones (they are pink), this will take less time than if you use raw (grey) ones. If you started with raw prawns, check they are cooked through.

4. Squeeze over the lemon juice and season with pepper to taste.

5. Serve divided among four bowls and scatter with parsley.

BREAKFAST

Caramelised banana and cocoa nib porridge

Breakfast really is the most important meal of the day, and porridge can be a great way to get yourself going. The oats are full of slow-release energy, and the bananas give you some important fruit and natural sweetness.

Under 400 calories

1 tbsp unsalted butter	700ml milk
½ tsp grated nutmeg	120g rolled oats
½ tsp ground cinnamon	150g cocoa nibs
4 bananas, peeled and sliced into coins	

1. Start by caramelising the bananas. In a small frying pan over a medium heat, add the butter and spices and heat until the butter is melted. If the sauce starts to bubble, turn the heat down, as you don't want it to burn.

2. Add the banana coins and stir to coat in the butter-spice mix. Fry the bananas for about 1 minute on each side, flipping them carefully so they don't fall apart.

3. Meanwhile, in a separate pan, make the porridge. Heat the milk and oats together over a low heat, stirring constantly, until the oats have absorbed all the milk.

4. Divide the oats among four bowls, top with the bananas and cocoa nibs to serve.

LUNCH

Aubergine, sweetcorn and avocado wraps

When you are trying to make nutritious, easy lunches it is really helpful to try to use up ingredients from meals on previous days. That's why this wrap uses the aubergines from Monday – less time spent preparing lunch means you might have more time to enjoy it!

Under 600 calories

Aubergines (leftover from
  Monday night)
1 x 330g tin of sweetcorn,
  rinsed and drained
2 avocados, halved, stoned
  and sliced

100g soured cream
150g mature Cheddar, grated
4 wholewheat tortilla wraps

1. Pile all the ingredients into the centre of each of the tortilla wraps.

2. Fold one side of the tortilla wrap in, then the opposite side. These will form the 'ends' that will stop the contents spilling out. Wrap the final two opposing sides in towards each other and enjoy.

DINNER

Salmon tacos

Salmon is a good source of heart-healthy omega 3 fats and protein. It is recommended you have at least one portion of oily fish per week, and salmon counts as one of them! This recipe is a real crowdpleaser, as everyone gets to make their own taco. The mashed avocado, tomato salsa, salmon and tacos are served separately in bowls on the table for everyone to help themselves.

550 calories

4 salmon fillets (approx. 500g)
2 tbsp olive oil
1 avocado, halved and stoned
Juice of 1 lime
1 tbsp olive oil
Chilli flakes, to taste

6 ripe tomatoes, roughly
   chopped
1 red onion, thinly sliced
Small handful of coriander,
   finely chopped
8 hard-shell tacos

1. Preheat the oven to 220°C/200°C fan/425°F/gas mark 7.

2. Place the salmon fillets in a baking dish, drizzle over the olive oil and bake in the oven for 20 minutes, until cooked through.

3. Scoop the flesh out of the avocado halves and mash it with the lime juice, olive oil and chilli flakes, then set aside in a bowl.

4. Mix together the tomatoes, red onion and coriander in a bowl, then set aside.

5. Heat the taco shells according to the packet instructions.

6. Serve the salmon, avocado, tomato salsa and taco shells separately on the table, allowing everyone to fill their own.

Get ahead

Tomorrow's breakfast takes a little longer to prepare, so I would suggest chopping the ingredients the day before and storing them in an airtight container in the fridge for the following morning, or preparing the beans and refrigerating them overnight.

Thursday

BREAKFAST

Healthy beans on toast

Beans on toast are, in my opinion, one of the ultimate comfort foods that I associate with my childhood. Beans are a great source of soluble fibre and protein, but traditional tinned 'baked beans' are often high in sugar and salt. This homemade version is a much healthier option.

400 calories

---

1 tbsp olive oil
1 pepper, deseeded and diced
1 red onion, diced
1 garlic clove, minced
2 tsp paprika
2 x 400g tins of chopped
   tomatoes

2 tbsp balsamic vinegar
2 x 400g tins of butter beans,
   rinsed and drained
4 slices of sourdough
Butter, for spreading

---

1. In a saucepan, heat the olive oil, then add the pepper and onion and fry until soft, about 5 minutes.

2. Add the garlic and paprika and cook for another 2 minutes.

3. Add the chopped tomatoes and balsamic vinegar, and simmer gently for another 15 minutes. At this stage, the sauce should be nice and thick.

4. Add the butter beans and cook until they are heated through, 3–4 minutes.

5. Toast the bread and spread with butter. Spoon over the baked beans to serve.

LUNCH

Nutty kale and chorizo salad with sriracha

This salad is a great texture combination of juicy chorizo, crunchy almonds and fibrous kale. The sriracha gives it a delicious spicy 'kick' – you can add more if you really want to heat it up!

Under 350 calories

1 tbsp olive oil
300g kale, tough stalks
   discarded, leaves chopped
   into bite-sized pieces
100g chorizo (leftover from
   Tuesday's dinner)

100g flaked almonds
Drizzle of sriracha
Juice of 1 lemon
Salt and pepper, to taste

1. Heat the olive oil in a large pan (big enough to contain all
   the kale) set over a medium heat. Add the kale and stir-fry
   for about 1 minute, until all the kale is coated in the hot oil.
   Put a small amount of water in the bottom of the pan (about
   4 tablespoons) and put the lid on the pan so the kale can
   steam. Leave to cook for about 5 minutes, until the kale
   is soft.

2. Remove the lid from the pan and cook until most of the water
   has evaporated – this prevents the kale becoming soggy.

3. Whilst still on the heat, stir the chorizo and almonds into the
   kale.

4. Dress the kale with the sriracha and lemon juice and season
   with salt and pepper. Stir well to coat then divide among four
   bowls to serve.

DINNER

Sweet potato burgers with a melting goat's cheese centre

This is one of my go-to recipes for cooking to impress even the most dedicated of meat-lovers. Lots of people are choosing to cook and eat less meat, but there are also still those who don't believe a meal without meat is a meal at all. It is so important to understand that whilst meat can make a valuable contribution to the diet, focusing on fruits, vegetables and healthy carbs is essential.

Under 550 calories

FOR THE BURGERS
2 sweet potatoes
1 red onion, roughly chopped
2 tsp ground cumin
1 tsp chilli flakes
2 tsp ground coriander
200g dried breadcrumbs
2 small goat's cheese rounds
Plain flour, for dusting

1 tsp olive oil

TO SERVE
1 x 100g rocket
1 tsp balsamic vinegar
1 tbsp olive oil
4 wholemeal burger buns,
   sliced in half

Get ahead

Breakfast tomorrow takes a few minutes of preparation tonight, to make sure you get the best flavour and texture in your chia pudding. Friday's dinner also benefits from a bit of forethought – the chicken needs to be marinated, and doing this in advance will really enhance the flavours.

1. Preheat the oven to 200°C/180°C fan/400°F/gas mark 6.

2. Prick the sweet potato skins and place on a baking tray. Bake for 15 minutes, before scattering the red onion around the sweet potatoes, then bake for a further 30 minutes, until the onion is soft.

3. Slice the sweet potatoes in half and scoop out the flesh, discarding the skins. Put the flesh into a blender with the red onion, cumin, chilli flakes and coriander. Blend until smooth.

4. Add the breadcrumbs to the mix. At this point it should start to feel a bit firmer. If it is still quite runny, add more breadcrumbs.

5. Cut each of the small goat's cheeses in half, so you have four pieces – one for each centre. Taking it in your hands, pat the sweet potato mix around the goat's cheese, so that you shape them into burgers and completely encase the cheese. It is really important to do this properly, otherwise the cheese will leak out during cooking as it melts.

6. Dust each burger with plain flour on each side.

7. Heat the olive oil in a frying pan, and fry the burgers for 5–7 minutes each side, until the burgers are golden brown on the outside. Careful when you 'flip' the burgers – make sure they don't fall apart.

8. Dress the rocket with balsamic vinegar and olive oil. Serve the burgers in the buns, with the side salad.

Friday

BREAKFAST

Raspberry, almond and mint chia pudding

This is a delicious, fresh twist on a chia pudding. The almonds give it some delicious 'crunch' and the raspberries add a lovely sweetness.

Under 400 calories

750ml hazelnut milk	200g raspberries
270g chia seeds	100g flaked almonds
1 tsp vanilla extract	Mint leaves, torn

1. Combine the hazelnut milk, chia seeds and vanilla extract in a jar or bowl and set in the fridge for 15 minutes, then remove and mix again. Cover the bowl or jar with a lid or cling film and return to the fridge overnight.

2. In the morning, remove the chia pudding from the fridge, divide among four bowls, top with the raspberries, flaked almonds and torn mint leaves and serve.

LUNCH

Soft cheese and roasted cherry tomato tartine

I really like the texture and flavour of cherry tomatoes with creamy soft cheese. For this recipe you roast the cherry tomatoes first, but if you are short of time you can use them raw.

350 calories

250g cherry tomatoes, cut in half
1 tbsp olive oil
4 slices of sourdough bread

150g soft cheese with garlic
Small handful of basil, leaves torn and stalks discarded

1. Preheat the oven to 200°C/180°C fan/400°F/gas mark 6.

2. Place the cherry tomatoes in a baking dish, pour over the olive oil and make sure they are all well coated. Bake for 20 minutes, until soft.

3. Toast the sourdough.

4. Spread each piece of toast with soft cheese, then pile it high with the cherry tomatoes and basil.

Tip: If you are making this recipe in advance to eat later (such as to take to work or school), keep the toast separate and assemble everything at the last minute to prevent the toast going soggy. Equally, you can leave the bread untoasted and make a sandwich (this might be easiest if you are making it for children who are taking it to school for lunch).

DINNER

Chicken, sweet potato and tarragon traybake

Traybakes are a really quick way to make a delicious meal. The meat juices help to cook the vegetables around the meat, giving them a delicious, sweet flavour. And, to top it off, there is very little washing-up! If you can marinate the chicken ahead of time, do so because the flavours will penetrate the chicken breasts better. I often do this the night before and refrigerate the chicken overnight. I've left the sweet potatoes unpeeled as this adds flavour and texture, as well as fibre and some vitamins. But you can peel them if you prefer!

450 calories

2 tbsp English mustard
1 tbsp olive oil
Zest and juice of 1 lemon
Salt and pepper, to taste
Small bunch of fresh tarragon, finely chopped

8 chicken thighs, skin on
3 sweet potatoes, cut into chunks
1 white onion, cut into eight wedges
300g green beans, trimmed

1. Preheat the oven to 200°C/180°C fan/400°F/gas mark 6.

2. Whisk the mustard, olive oil, lemon zest and juice, salt, pepper and tarragon together in a small bowl. Pour over the chicken thighs in a large bowl and leave to marinade for at least half an hour, or overnight if you can.

3. In a roasting dish, place the sweet potatoes, onion wedges and chicken thighs with their marinade. Mix well, so that the sweet potato and onion is also coated in the marinade.

4. Roast for 45 minutes to 1 hour, until the chicken is golden brown and the vegetables are soft.

5. Just before serving, steam the green beans. To do this, put the beans in the top half of a double boiler, with about 2.5cm of water in the bottom half of the double boiler, and steam for about 5 minutes. If you don't have a double boiler, boiling the green beans is fine.

6. Serve the chicken and vegetables with the beans alongside.

Recipes: Week 3

N.B. Each meal serves four people
unless otherwise stated.

MENU

	Breakfast	Lunch	Dinner
Saturday	Healthy breakfast muffins	Spanish omelette	Harissa-baked chicken with flatbreads and salad
Sunday	Spicy baked eggs with chorizo and halloumi	Spicy shredded Vietnamese chicken salad	Beef massaman curry
Monday	Apple and sultana bircher muesli	Chicken, feta and lettuce pitta pockets	Chicken laksa
Tuesday	Egg in a cup	Avocado, mango and cucumber salad	Beef and lentil cottage pie with roasted broccoli

	Breakfast	Lunch	Dinner
Wednesday	Mango and coconut bircher muesli	Roasted broccoli and goat's cheese tartine	Ginger and soy steamed sea bass
Thursday	Egg-in-a-hole with cherry tomato salsa	Beetroot and feta wrap	Sweet potato dhal with toasted coconut flakes
Friday	Creamy porridge with berry jam	Cucumber, cream cheese and dill bagels	Grilled tuna steaks with a cherry tomato salsa

SHOPPING LIST

Carbohydrate

- ☐ 1.5kg waxy potatoes
- ☐ 4 wholemeal pitta breads
- ☐ 300g dried rice noodles
- ☐ 4 wholemeal wraps
- ☐ 4 plain bagels
- ☐ 4 flatbreads
- ☐ 2 sweet potatoes
- ☐ 4 wholemeal bread rolls

Dairy products

- ☐ 300ml 0% fat natural yoghurt
- ☐ 1 x 250g block halloumi
- ☐ 600g Greek yoghurt
- ☐ 300g low-fat crème fraîche
- ☐ 550g feta cheese
- ☐ 1 x 280g tub of cream cheese
- ☐ 300g soft goat's cheese
- ☐ 3 pints of milk

Meat, fish and meat alternatives

- ☐ 300g chorizo
- ☐ 10 skinless chicken breasts
- ☐ 600g beef stewing steak
- ☐ 300g lean beef mince
- ☐ 300ml fresh beef stock
- ☐ 4 sea bass fillets
- ☐ 4 tuna steaks
- ☐ 18 eggs (plus 5 leftover from last week)

Fruits/vegetables

- ☐ 1 banana
- ☐ 3 red onions
- ☐ 1 bulb garlic
- ☐ 2 large eating apples
- ☐ 200g baby spinach leaves
- ☐ 400g frozen mango chunks
- ☐ 500g strawberries (fresh or frozen)
- ☐ 2 red peppers
- ☐ 1 carrot

- [ ] 4 white onions
- [ ] 4 romaine lettuces
- [ ] 9 limes
- [ ] 1 bunch of spring onions
- [ ] 350g mangetout
- [ ] 400g Tenderstem broccoli
- [ ] 2 lemons
- [ ] 100g rocket
- [ ] 2 beetroots
- [ ] 2 avocados
- [ ] 2 cucumbers
- [ ] 2 heads of pak choi
- [ ] 550g cherry tomatoes

Other – dried larder foods

- [ ] 2 x 400g tins of chopped tomatoes
- [ ] Massaman curry paste
- [ ] 2 x 400ml tins of coconut milk
- [ ] 1 x 400g tin of ready-cooked Puy lentils
- [ ] 1 x 250g packet of ready-cooked Puy lentils
- [ ] 300g red split lentils

Fresh herbs

- [ ] Root ginger
- [ ] Coriander
- [ ] Mint
- [ ] Dill
- [ ] Parsley
- [ ] 2 lemongrass stalks

Dried fruits and nuts:

- [ ] 150g flame raisins
- [ ] 200g sultanas*
- [ ] 100g dried apricots
- [ ] 150g linseeds
- [ ] 100g dessicated coconut
- [ ] 50g flaked almonds*
- [ ] 250g unsalted peanuts
- [ ] 100g coconut flakes

*You should have leftovers of these from previous weeks.

BREAKFAST

Healthy breakfast muffins

Muffins are traditionally very high in fat and sugar, however, much of the moisture in the batter here comes from yoghurt, which makes these much lower in fat than their shop-bought counterparts. This recipe makes more muffins than you need, but they keep well in the freezer – just get them out the night before for an on-the-go breakfast.

Makes about 12 muffins (recommended serving size = 2 muffins).
150 calories per muffin

1 egg, beaten	1 tsp ground cinnamon
300ml 0% fat natural yoghurt	150g flame raisins (the big juicy ones!)
100ml skimmed milk	
1 tsp vanilla extract	100g dried apricots, chopped
1 banana, mashed	30g rolled oats
300g plain flour	50g flaked almonds
2 tsp bicarbonate of soda	

1. Preheat the oven to 180°C/160°C fan/350°F/gas mark 4 and line a 12-hole muffin tin with muffin cases, or just grease the holes in the muffin tin.

2. Combine the wet ingredients – egg, yoghurt, skimmed milk, vanilla extract and banana – together thoroughly in a large bowl.

3. Add the dry ingredients – flour, bicarbonate of soda, cinnamon, dried fruits, oats and almonds – and stir to combine.

4. Divide the mixture among the paper cases or muffin tin holes.

5. Bake for about 20 minutes, until the muffin tops are golden brown – if you insert a skewer in the middle, it should come out clean.

LUNCH

Spanish omelette

This recipe is a real lunchtime and quick evening staple in my house. Frittatas in general are a great way of using up any leftovers. Eggs are a very protein-rich way of holding all the other delicious ingredients together. I've made one here with potatoes and chorizo, like the traditional Spanish omelette, but lots of other fillings work well, too.

453 calories

6 eggs	1 white onion, finely diced
300ml low-fat crème fraîche	1 red pepper, deseeded and cut
Pinch of pepper	into small pieces
300g waxy potatoes, cut in	100g chorizo, cut into small
half	pieces
1 tsp olive oil	

Get ahead

Chicken will take on stronger flavours from a marinade if you can prepare it in advance. So I would recommend making tonight's dinner at least a few hours ahead, marinating the meat in the fridge. If you are not able to do this, even leaving it for half an hour will make a difference. You could also prepare the marinade for Sunday lunch at the same time, too.

1. Whisk the eggs and crème fraîche together, add a pinch of pepper, then set aside.

2. Boil the potatoes for about 10 minutes, until soft. Drain and set aside to cool.

3. Once the potatoes are cool, slice them into roughly 0.5cm-thick slices.

4. In a large deep ovenproof frying pan set over a medium heat add the olive oil and cook the onion and red pepper. When the vegetables are soft, add the chorizo and cook for a further few minutes, until the chorizo is soft, too. Add the potatoes and stir gently to mix – be gentle, you don't want the potato to break up.

5. Pour over the egg mixture, then cook for a few minutes, until just beginning to set at the base of the pan.

6. Heat the grill to medium and cook the omelette for about 15 minutes, until the eggs are well set. If you don't have a grill, cook the omelette in an oven preheated to 220°C/200°C fan/425°F/gas mark 7 for 10 minutes.

DINNER

Harissa-baked chicken with flatbreads and salad

The marinade for this salad is so quick and easy to make; you just put all the ingredients in a blender. However, if you don't have a blender to hand, chopping the herbs and stirring all the ingredients together will do just as well. It is also delicious for other meat, such as lamb, or even on tofu for a vegetarian alternative. This dish is a lovely combination of chicken and lots of delicious, crunchy vegetables.

490 calories

FOR THE CHICKEN
4 tbsp harissa paste
4 tbsp olive oil
Handful of coriander leaves
Juice of 2 limes
Pinch of pepper
1 garlic clove

6 skinless chicken breasts

TO SERVE
4 flatbreads
1 romaine lettuce, leaves cut
    into strips

1. Preheat the oven to 220°C/200°C fan/425°F/gas mark 7.

2. Start by making the marinade for the chicken. In a blender, combine the harissa paste, olive oil, coriander, lime juice, pepper and garlic. Blend until smooth.

3. Place the chicken breasts in an ovenproof dish and pour over the marinade. Leave to marinate for at least 30 minutes, but ideally overnight.

4. Bake the chicken in the marinade in the oven for 25–30 minutes, until the marinade is bubbling and the chicken is cooked through – the meat should be white and the juices run clear when it is poked with a skewer or a knife.

5. Heat the flatbreads for about 5 minutes in the oven, just as the chicken has finished cooking.

6. Set aside two chicken breasts, allow them to cool before covering and refrigerating them. (These are for lunch on Monday.)

7. Serve the chicken and flatbreads on plates with the lettuce, drizzling any remaining marinade over the lettuce as a dressing.

Sunday

BREAKFAST

Spicy baked eggs with chorizo and halloumi

This recipe is a spicy twist on a breakfast staple – eggs. Eggs are high in protein, which is important for repairing damaged cells in your body and keeping you full – making them a great breakfast food! The halloumi and chorizo give this recipe lots of flavour and texture.

597 calories

1 tbsp olive oil	2 x 400g tins of chopped tomatoes
2 red onions, chopped	200g chorizo, diced
1 garlic clove, minced	1 x 250g block of halloumi, cut into small pieces
2 tsp chilli flakes, or more, to taste	4 eggs
Small bunch of coriander, stalks and leaves chopped separately	Pepper, to taste

1. Over a medium heat, heat the olive oil in a wide frying pan that has a lid. When the oil is hot, add the red onions and garlic and cook until tender, about 5 minutes.

2. Add the chilli flakes and coriander stalks and cook for a further minute or two, until aromatic.

3. Add the chopped tomatoes and simmer for about 10 minutes, until the sauce has thickened.

4. Add the chorizo and halloumi to the tomato sauce and stir thoroughly.

5. Make four small 'wells' in the tomato sauce and crack an egg into each one. Put the lid on the saucepan and cook for a further 5 minutes – popping on the lid will allow the eggs to slightly steam, so they cook evenly.

6. To serve, sprinkle over the coriander leaves and crack over some pepper.

LUNCH

Spicy shredded Vietnamese chicken salad

This salad is so fresh and crunchyand is packed with vitamins and minerals from the rainbow of vegetables, and protein from the peanuts and chicken. I love the zesty chicken sauce here – adding fish sauce gives it that authentic Asian taste, while the sriracha adds a little heat. Feel free to add extra sriracha if you like your food really spicy!

464 calories

FOR THE CHICKEN

2 skinless chicken breasts, cut into strips

Juice of 3 limes

3 tbsp olive oil

3 tsp fish sauce

2 tbsp sriracha (or more, if you are feeling brave)

1 thumb-sized piece of root ginger, minced

1 garlic clove, minced

FOR THE SALAD

1 red pepper, deseeded and thinly sliced

1 carrot, peeled and sliced into matchsticks

1 romaine lettuce, thinly sliced

Small handful of mint, finely chopped

Small handful of coriander, finely chopped

200g unsalted peanuts, roughly chopped (some supermarkets sell these ready chopped in the baking section, so use these if you prefer)

1. Preheat the oven to 220°C/200°C fan/425°F/gas mark 7.

2. In a baking dish, place the chicken breasts and add in all the other ingredients. Stir well to combine.

3. Bake the chicken for 20 minutes, until the meat is white and the sauce is bubbling.

4. Combine all the salad ingredients together in a large bowl.

5. Add the chicken pieces to the salad and pour over the sauce to double up as a dressing.

DINNER

Beef massaman curry

Massaman curry is one of my absolute favourites – easy to make and really delicious. Because this curry has potatoes in it, you don't need extra carbs to make this into a hearty meal. I recommend having some veg on the side instead – such as steamed green beans – to balance it out.

539 calories

1 tsp olive oil
600g beef stewing steak, cut into bite-sized chunks
1 red onion, diced
4 tbsp massaman curry paste
1 tbsp tamarind paste
1 tsp chilli flakes
1 x 400ml tin of coconut milk
1 tbsp fish sauce
450g waxy potatoes, cut into bite-sized chunks
Juice of 1 lime

TO SERVE
50g unsalted peanuts, roughly chopped
Handful of coriander, finely chopped
3 spring onions, finely sliced

1. Preheat the oven to 200°C/180°C fan/400°F/gas mark 6.

2. Heat the olive oil in an ovenproof pan and add the beef and onion. Cook for 5–7 minutes, until the onion is soft and the beef is browned all over.

3. Add the curry paste, tamarind paste and chilli flakes and cook for a further 2 minutes, until aromatic.

4. Add the coconut milk, fish sauce, potatoes and lime juice to the pan. Bring to a gentle simmer, then put into the oven for 1½–2 hours, until the potatoes and beef are soft and the sauce is thick.

5. When the curry has finished cooking, divide among four bowls and top with the peanuts, coriander and spring onions.

Get ahead

Tomorrow morning's bircher muesli needs to be prepared in advance to give the oats enough time to soak up the yoghurt and milk and become really soft, so do this the night before and it'll be ready to go in the morning when you're in a rush.

BREAKFAST

Apple and sultana bircher muesli

Bircher muesli is a breakfast classic. It is also very quick to make; you can even make it in batches and keep in in the fridge. The oats make it high in soluble fibre and the Greek yoghurt is packed full of protein. You can flavour it with any fruit, nuts or spices you like, but this combination is a real winner.

479 calories

250g rolled oats
250g Greek yoghurt
250ml milk
2 tsp vanilla extract
1 thumb-sized piece of root
    ginger, grated

50g linseeds
200g flame raisins
1 tsp grated nutmeg
2 large apples, coarsely grated

1. Combine the oats, Greek yoghurt, milk, vanilla extract, ginger, linseeds, raisins and nutmeg in a large bowl, cover and leave in the fridge overnight.

2. In the morning, stir through the apple and divide among four bowls.

LUNCH

Chicken, feta and lettuce pitta pockets

Using leftovers makes for a very easy lunch – and here we're stuffing the chicken from Saturday's dinner into pitta breads to make a new and different meal with minimal effort. The creaminess of the feta really tops it off.

374 calories

4 wholemeal pitta breads
Unsalted butter, for spreading
2 harissa-baked chicken
    breasts (leftover from
    Saturday), finely sliced

1 romaine lettuce, finely sliced
150g feta cheese, crumbled

1. Toast the pitta breads, then slice them and open them out ready to fill.

2. Spread each pitta thinly inside with butter on one side, then stuff with the remaining ingredients.

DINNER

Chicken laksa

This aromatic Malaysian soup is packed full of chicken and rice noodles – it is a lovely, filling dish and is so easy to make for something with so much flavour.

2 skinless chicken breasts, cut into pieces
3cm piece of root ginger, sliced
Juice of 1 lime
2 lemongrass stalks, crushed
2 tbsp fish sauce
1 tbsp soy sauce
2 garlic cloves, minced
Handful of coriander, chopped (leaves and stalks kept separate)
1 tsp chilli flakes (or more, if you are feeling brave)
1 x 400ml tin of coconut milk
200g mangetout
300g dried rice noodles
200g baby spinach leaves
3 spring onions, sliced, to serve

1. In a large saucepan, place the chicken pieces, ginger, lime juice, lemongrass, fish sauce, soy sauce, garlic cloves, coriander stalks and chilli flakes. Cover with water and simmer for about 30 minutes, until the chicken is cooked through and falling apart.

2. Add the coconut milk and mangetout, then simmer until hot through, about 3 minutes.

3. Stir through the rice noodles and spinach leaves and cook until the spinach and noodles are soft.

4. To serve, divide among four bowls and top with spring onions and coriander.

Tuesday

BREAKFAST

Egg in a cup

This was my ultimate comfort food as a child. Extremely easy to make, totally delicious, and who doesn't love eating their food out of a mug?

315 calories

---

8 eggs

4 wholemeal bread rolls

50g unsalted butter, cut into
   small cubes

Salt and pepper, to taste

---

1. Gently lower the eggs into a pan of boiling water, using a spoon, and boil for 4 minutes.

2. Whilst the eggs are boiling, tear up the bread rolls and divide among four large mugs. Sprinkle the butter over the bread.

3. Remove the eggs from the boiling water. Crack the shell of the eggs all the way around, and using the back of a teaspoon, gently peel the shell from the eggs, discarding the shell. Spoon two eggs into each mug and mix around to make sure the bread is coated and the butter is melting.

4. Season and serve.

LUNCH

Avocado, mango and cucumber salad

This salad is really fresh-tasting, thanks in part to the zesty mango and lime combined with cool mint and cucumber. I like to use frozen mango, which I take out of the freezer and thaw overnight, as it is cheaper than fresh. If you would rather use fresh, use two mangoes instead.

416 calories

2 avocados, stoned and flesh
 cut into small chunks
150g frozen mango, thawed
1 romaine lettuce, shredded
½ cucumber, cut into small
 chunks
200g feta cheese, crumbled

1 x 250g packet of ready-
 cooked Puy lentils
Juice of 1 lime
2 tbsp olive oil
Pinch of chilli flakes
Pepper, to taste
Handful of mint, finely
 chopped

1. Mix the avocado, mango, lettuce, cucumber, feta and lentils together in a large bowl.

2. Pour over the lime juice and drizzle with the olive oil.

3. Add the chilli and pepper and toss until well combined. Serve divided among four bowls, with the mint scattered on top.

DINNER

Beef and lentil cottage pie with roasted broccoli

Adding in pulses, such as the lentils here, to dishes is a good way to get some low-fat, cheaper protein to replace some of the red meat. And, provided they are cooked in the right way, they make a delicious contribution to the recipe, too!

509 calories

FOR THE MASH TOPPING
750g waxy potatoes, peeled
  and chopped
50ml milk
75g unsalted butter

FOR THE MINCE FILLING
1 tbsp olive oil
1 white onion, finely chopped
1 garlic clove, minced
300g lean beef mince

2 tbsp tomato purée
1 x 400g tin of ready-cooked
  Puy lentils, rinsed and
  drained
300ml fresh beef stock

TO SERVE
400g Tenderstem broccoli
1 tbsp olive oil
1 tsp chilli flakes

Get ahead

Tomorrow's breakfast is another bircher muesli, also called 'overnight oats'. So the clue is in the name – it is best to start this the night before, cover it and leave it in the fridge.

1. Preheat the oven to 190°C/170°C fan/375°F/gas mark 5.

2. Start by making the mashed potato. In a saucepan of lightly salted water, boil the potatoes for about 15 minutes, until soft. You don't want to over-boil them, or the mash will be soggy.

3. Drain the potatoes, put them into a large bowl with the milk and butter and mash until completely smooth. If you want to, you can always use a food processor to make sure you get all the lumps out. Set the potato mash aside.

4. In a large pan, heat the oil and add the onion and garlic. Fry until soft, about 5 minutes. When the onion and garlic are soft, add the beef mince and fry for 5–10 minutes, until browned and cooked through.

5. Stir the tomato purée and lentils into the mince, then add the stock. Cover and simmer for about 20 minutes.

6. Transfer the mince to an ovenproof dish, then top with the mashed potato. Bake for about 30 minutes, until the mash is golden brown.

7. About 10 minutes before the cottage pie is ready, roast the broccoli. Put it into an ovenproof dish, drizzle with the olive oil and scatter with the chilli flakes, then roast in the oven alongside the pie for 10 minutes. When the broccoli is cooked through, set aside half for lunch on Wednesday.

8. Serve the cottage pie with the broccoli on the side.

BREAKFAST

Mango and coconut bircher muesli

If you ever wanted a breakfast that would make you feel like you are on holiday, this is it! I use frozen mango as it is often cheaper than fresh (and then you don't have to worry about it being in season!). Some people think that freezing fruits and vegetables reduces their nutritional value, but it actually does the opposite – it preserves them better.

469 calories

250g rolled oats	2 tsp vanilla extract
250g Greek yoghurt	250g frozen mango chunks
250ml milk	100g dessicated coconut

1. Combine the oats, Greek yoghurt, milk, vanilla extract and frozen mango chunks in a large bowl, cover and leave in the fridge overnight.

2. In the morning, divide among four bowls and scatter over the coconut just before serving.

LUNCH

Roasted broccoli and goat's cheese tartine

This tartine is so pretty, thanks in part to the roasted broccoli from last night's dinner. Roasting broccoli helps to preserve its vitamins, which can be washed away when boiling. It is also delicious and gives a crunchier texture, which goes well with the cream cheese used here.

376 calories

---

4 slices of wholemeal
   sourdough
300g soft goat's cheese
200g roasted broccoli

(leftover from Tuesday
   night's dinner)
Salt and pepper, to taste

---

1. Toast the sourdough.

2. Spread each piece of toast thickly with goat's cheese, then pile them high with broccoli. Sprinkle with salt and pepper to serve.

Wednesday

DINNER

Ginger and soy steamed sea bass

I try to use wholegrain carbohydrates (which are often brown) rather than refined ones (which are normally white), because of their higher fibre content. I love brown rice – it has a certain nuttiness to it, which gives it a great texture – but you do need to be a bit more patient as it is quite slow to cook. For this recipe you will need a steamer – if you don't already own one they are well worth the investment, as they are a very healthy way to cook vegetables.

340 calories

360g brown rice	2 tbsp sesame oil
4 sea bass fillets	4 tbsp soy sauce
150g mangetout	Pinch of chilli flakes
Thumb-sized piece of root ginger, grated	2 heads of pak choi, cut into quarters
2 garlic cloves, minced	Handful of coriander, chopped

1. Cook the brown rice according to the packet instructions.

2. Line the top of the steamer with tin foil and place the sea bass (skin side up to prevent it drying out) and mangetout inside. It doesn't matter if they overlap slightly during cooking.

3. Combine the ginger, garlic, sesame oil, soy sauce and chilli flakes together, then pour everything over the fish.

4. Cover the steamer with a lid and steam the fish for 2 minutes, then add the pak choi to the steamer and cook for another 6 minutes.

5. Serve the brown rice in the centre of the plate. Lay over the fish (gently, so you don't break it up), then top with veggies. Pour any leftover juices over the top and scatter with coriander.

BREAKFAST

Egg-in-a-hole with cherry tomato salsa

Egg in a hole is an easy way to cook fried eggs – and very pretty, too! If you want to get really creative, you can use different-shaped cookie cutters. The tomato salsa means it counts as one of your five-a-day.

50g unsalted butter, softened
4 slices of sourdough brown
   bread (from the freezer)
4 eggs
350g cherry tomatoes, cut in
   half

Small bunch of parsley, finely
   chopped
Pepper, to serve

1. Butter each slice of bread on both sides then cut a hole out of the middle, roughly the size of a fried egg. You can toast these centres while everything else is cooking, to munch on as a tasty snack while you wait!

2. Place each slice of bread in a frying pan over a low–medium heat.

3. Cook the bread for about 2 minutes, then flip over. Crack the egg in the middle of the hole and cook for about 3 minutes, until the egg is firm and cooked through. Carefully flip the bread again, so that the egg can cook on both sides.

4. Remove from the pan and scatter each 'egg-in-a-hole' with cherry tomatoes, parsley and pepper, then serve immediately.

Thursday

LUNCH

Beetroot and feta wrap

Beetroot and feta is a classic, tried-and-tested (and well-loved!) combination. It makes a great lunch – the beetroot is a beautiful colour, so we can eat with our eyes as well as our stomachs!

343 calories

200g feta cheese	Pinch of pepper
Zest and juice of 1 lemon	Pinch of chilli flakes
1 garlic clove	4 wholemeal wraps
1 tsp olive oil	100g rocket
Small handful of mint	2 beetroots, peeled and grated

1. In a blender, combine the feta, lemon zest and juice, garlic, olive oil, mint, pepper and chilli until smooth.

2. Spread each wrap with the feta dip, then pile on the rocket and beetroot. If you, like me, don't like to make a mess, make sure you fold the wrap up well to stop it 'exploding' whilst eating. You can do this by folding each end in first, then rolling it up.

Thursday

DINNER

Sweet potato dhal with toasted coconut flakes

Dhal, a traditional Indian curry made with lentils, is a great source of healthy plant protein and fibre, with very little fat. This dhal is easy to make, and full of delicious, aromatic spices.

450 calories

1 tbsp olive oil
2 white onions, finely diced
2 thumb-sized pieces of root
  ginger, finely chopped
4 garlic cloves, finely chopped
1 tsp chilli flakes (more if you
  like!)
3 tsp mustard seeds
1 tsp cumin seeds
2 sweet potatoes, peeled and
  cut into bite-sized chunks
300g red split lentils
900ml water
100g coconut flakes

Handful of coriander, finely
  chopped
Zest and juice of 1 lime

FOR THE RAITA
100g Greek yoghurt
½ tsp ground cumin
½ cucumber, grated
Handful of coriander, finely
  chopped
2 spring onions, finely chopped
Handful of mint, finely
  chopped

1. Heat the olive oil in a large saucepan over a medium heat, then add the onions, ginger and garlic and fry for about 5 minutes, until soft. Add the chilli flakes, mustard and cumin seeds and cook for another few minutes, until aromatic.

2. Add the sweet potatoes and lentils, cover with water and simmer for about 35 minutes, until the lentils have absorbed all the water. Then mash everything together roughly with a potato masher.

3. While the dhal is cooking, make the raita by combining all the ingredients.

4. In a shallow frying pan over a medium heat, dry-fry the coconut flakes.

5. Serve the dhal with the raita, coconut flakes, coriander and lime zest scattered over. Finally, squeeze over the lime juice.

Get ahead

The berry jam for tomorrow's breakfast contains chia seeds, so just like the chia puddings last week, you need to prepare these in advance to allow the chia seeds to expand and form a jelly-like texture (perfect sugar-free jam!).

BREAKFAST

Creamy porridge with berry jam

Jam is really just sugar held together with a bit of fruit, so you might be surprised to see it in a low-sugar cookbook. However, substitute the sugar for chia seeds (which are low in sugar and high in soluble fibre) and you have a great added-sugar-free alternative! You should make the jam the night before you need it, because the chia seeds need time to swell and absorb some of the fruit juices. You will have lots of leftover jam, so keep some in the fridge in a sterile jar for later – it will keep for about a week.

458 calories

FOR THE JAM	FOR THE PORRIDGE
500g strawberries, fresh or frozen	120g rolled oats
½ tsp vanilla extract	700ml milk
30g chia seeds	100g linseeds

N.B. – to sterilise the jar:
Wash the jar and its lid in hot soapy water then stand both upside down in a roasting tin while they're still wet. Put the tin in an oven preheated to 170°C/150°C fan/325°F/gas mark 3 for about 15 minutes. Use the jar immediately.

1. In a small saucepan, gently heat the strawberries for 5–10 minutes, until thawed and beginning to soften. If using fresh strawberries, this should happen after 3–5 minutes. When soft, mash them with a fork or potato masher. Add the vanilla extract and chia seeds, and stir over the heat for a further few minutes. Remove the saucepan from the heat and tip the jam into a sterilised jar, seal, and, once cool, store in the fridge.

2. To make the porridge, heat the oats, milk and linseeds together over a low heat for about 5 minutes, stirring constantly, until the oats have absorbed all the milk.

3. Serve the porridge topped with 2 tablespoons of chia jam per portion (or more, if you like!).

LUNCH

Cucumber, cream cheese and dill bagels

450 calories

---

4 plain bagels, cut in half
1 x 280g tub of cream cheese
½ cucumber, finely sliced

Handful of dill, finely chopped
Pepper, to taste

---

1. Toast the bagels.

2. Spread each half of the bagels with cream cheese, fill with
   cucumber slices, dill and a little pepper, then sandwich back
   together to serve.

DINNER

Grilled tuna steaks with a cherry tomato salsa

Tuna is a really good source of heart-healthy omega 3 fatty acids and lean protein. I would always recommend that you source it carefully, though, due to the environmental impact that poor fishing practices can have on tuna populations and other marine life that share the same habitat. I love this recipe, as the fresh salsa complements the meaty tuna so well. It is important that you do not overcook the tuna – it is best served slightly 'pink' in the middle; the resting time is also important to allow the muscle fibres to relax to prevent the meat being too tough.

450 calories

4 tuna steaks
1 tsp olive oil
200g brown rice

FOR THE SALSA
½ cucumber, diced
200g cherry tomatoes,
   cut in half

Handful of parsley, finely
   chopped
Pinch of chilli flakes
Juice of 1 lemon
1 tsp olive oil

1. Rub the tuna steaks with the olive oil and set aside.

2. Cook the rice according to the packet instructions.

3. To make the salsa, mix all ingredients together.

4. About 10 minutes before the rice has finished cooking, heat a shallow frying pan over a medium heat. Fry each tuna steak for about 2 minutes each side, before removing from the pan and setting aside for 5 minutes to rest.

5. Serve the rice with the tuna steaks on top, each topped with salsa.

Get ahead

If you can, I would recommend making Saturday's breakfast in advance. The recipe makes a large batch, which will keep very well in an airtight container for a few weeks, so this can be made the night before or even the week before!

Recipes: Week 4

N.B. Each meal serves four people
unless otherwise stated.

MENU

	Breakfast	Lunch	Dinner
Saturday	Buttermilk rusks with cranberries and pistachios	Tom yum soup	Pesto and chicken crumble with green salad
Sunday	Green mushroom, and ricotta crêpes	One-pot roast chicken	Sundried tomato and mozzarella tart with rocket and walnut pesto
Monday	Apricot, blueberry and hazelnut chia pudding	Peach, mozzarella and Parma ham salad	Harissa-marinated lamb kebabs with Greek salad
Tuesday	Menemen	Pesto chickpea salad with cherry tomatoes	Chicken skewers with rainbow slaw and warm pittas

	Breakfast	**Lunch**	**Dinner**
Wednesday	Porridge with rhubarb and ginger	Artichoke, broad bean and feta salad	Smoked mackerel kedgeree
Thursday	Spicy scrambled eggs	Roast vegetable and goat's cheese frittata	Asparagus and lemon pearl barley risotto
Friday	Carrot and sultana drop scones	Ricotta, pea and asparagus tartine	Hake with hasselback potatoes and braised veggies

SHOPPING LIST

Carbohydrate
- [ ] 250g ciabatta bread
- [ ] 8 wholemeal pittas
- [ ] 1 sheet all-butter puff pastry
- [ ] 300g pearl barley
- [ ] 400g couscous

Dairy products
- [ ] 400ml buttermilk
- [ ] 400g ricotta cheese
- [ ] 425g mozzarella
- [ ] 300g Parmesan cheese
- [ ] 3 pints of milk
- [ ] 250g tub of mascarpone
- [ ] 450g feta cheese
- [ ] 300ml low-fat crème fraîche
- [ ] 150g hard goat's cheese
- [ ] 200g Greek yoghurt
- [ ] 250g plain yoghurt

Meat, fish and meat alternatives
- [ ] 5 skinless chicken breasts
- [ ] 200g cooked prawns
- [ ] 1.4l fresh chicken stock
- [ ] 100g Parma ham
- [ ] 300g cooked chicken, skinless
- [ ] 1 medium-sized chicken (approx. 1.5kg)
- [ ] 300g smoked mackerel fillets
- [ ] 400g lamb steak
- [ ] 4 hake fillets
- [ ] 100g bacon lardons
- [ ] 22 eggs

Fruits/vegetables
- [ ] 400g spinach leaves
- [ ] 7 lemons
- [ ] 400g chestnut mushrooms
- [ ] 6 limes
- [ ] 4 fresh peaches
- [ ] Small punnet of berries (optional)
- [ ] 600g rocket
- [ ] 1 romaine lettuce
- [ ] 1 bulb garlic
- [ ] 9 carrots

- ☐ Bunch of spring onions
- ☐ 1 white cabbage
- ☐ 200g parsnips
- ☐ 100g beetroot
- ☐ 800g cherry tomatoes
- ☐ 3 white onions
- ☐ 500g asparagus
- ☐ 1 fennel bulb
- ☐ 7 celery sticks
- ☐ 4 red peppers
- ☐ 5 red onions
- ☐ 8 large plum tomatoes
- ☐ 2 cucumbers
- ☐ 1 aubergine
- ☐ 1 courgette
- ☐ 3 red chillies
- ☐ 400g rhubarb
- ☐ 200g blueberries
- ☐ 300g green beans

Other – dried larder foods

- ☐ 190g jar of green pesto
- ☐ 1 x 225g jar of sundried tomatoes
- ☐ Small jar of black olives
- ☐ 2 x 400g tins of chickpeas

- ☐ 300g jar of artichoke hearts
- ☐ 10g dried yeast

Fresh herbs

- ☐ Chives
- ☐ Coriander
- ☐ Ginger
- ☐ Mint
- ☐ Basil
- ☐ Parsley
- ☐ 1 lemongrass stalk
- ☐ 3 kaffir lime leaves
- ☐ Root ginger

Dried fruits and nuts

- ☐ 200g sultanas*
- ☐ 200g dried cranberries
- ☐ 100g dried apricots
- ☐ 150g walnuts
- ☐ 200g pistachios*
- ☐ 50g hazelnuts*

*You should have leftovers of these from previous weeks.

Saturday

BREAKFAST

Buttermilk rusks with cranberries and pistachios

Rusks are traditional South African breakfast biscuits, which are double-baked so that they are very crunchy and crumbly. They make great on-the-go breakfasts as they are lower in sugar than traditional biscuits. They are also delicious dunked in tea!

Makes about 15 rusks
275 calories per rusk

400ml buttermilk	700g plain flour
100g unsalted butter, melted	200g dried cranberries
10g dried yeast (2 sachets)	200g pistachios, roughly
½ tsp salt	chopped
½ bicarbonate of soda	

1. Preheat the oven to 180°C/160°C fan/350°F/gas mark 4.

2. In a large mixing bowl, combine the buttermilk and melted butter. Stir in the yeast, until it starts to bubble gently.

3. Add the salt and bicarbonate of soda and mix well.

4. Add the flour, a small amount at a time, and stir until it forms a dough.

5. Add the cranberries and pistachios and mix well into the dough.

6. Cover the dough with a damp cloth and leave to prove in a warm area for about 1 hour.

7. Pour the dough into a baking dish, and bake for about 35 minutes, until golden brown and cooked through. It should still be quite soft to the touch.

8. Remove from the oven, and leave the mixture to cool completely, then slice into 26 evenly sized rusks.

9. Turn the temperature of the oven down to 100°C/80°C fan/200°F/gas mark ¼. Lay the sliced rusks out flat on baking sheets, making sure they don't touch, and bake in the oven for about 8 hours. Some people recommend doing this overnight, but if you worry about the safety of having the oven on overnight I would recommend doing this during the day.

LUNCH

Tom yum soup

Tom yum is a traditional Asian soup – it's a thin chicken broth filled with chicken, prawn and lots of vegetables, and it is one of my absolute favourite lunches! I like mine quite spicy (which is more traditional), but go light on the chilli if you are not feeling so brave. I would recommend either making the chicken stock or buying it fresh from a supermarket instead of using stock cubes – it gives the soup a much better flavour.

206 calories

1.4 litres fresh chicken stock
1 lemongrass stalk, bruised and cut into large pieces
Small bunch of coriander, leaves and stalks chopped separately
3 kaffir lime leaves
Juice of 2 limes

3 red chillies, finely chopped
75ml Thai fish sauce
100g fresh root ginger, grated
2 skinless chicken breasts, cut into small chunks
200g cooked prawns (not frozen)
150g spinach leaves

1. In a large saucepan, bring the chicken stock to the boil.

2. Add the lemongrass, coriander stalks, lime leaves, lime juice, chillies, fish sauce and ginger, reduce the heat and simmer for 15–20 minutes to allow the flavours to really infuse the stock.

3. Add the chicken chunks and cook for about 5 minutes, until cooked through.

4. Add the prawns and spinach and cook until hot through. Ladle into four bowls and serve, sprinkled with coriander leaves.

DINNER

Pesto and chicken crumble with green salad

I love this recipe – it really is one of my go-to dinners. It is fast to make and the creamy pesto and mascarpone sauce is so tasty. By packing it full of peas and spinach, it is also healthier than it tastes.

For this recipe you make far more dressing than you need, so save it in a clean container in the fridge to use in salads later in the week (see page 200).

552 calories

FOR THE SALAD AND
DRESSING
Juice of 1 lemon
30ml balsamic vinegar
100ml olive oil
2 tsp English mustard
1 romaine lettuce, shredded

FOR THE TOPPING
40g unsalted butter, softened
75g plain flour
25g rolled oats
50g Parmesan cheese, grated

FOR THE CHICKEN
190g jar of green pesto
250g tub of mascarpone
250ml water
200g spinach
250g frozen peas
Small bunch of basil and mint,
    chopped
Splash of milk
300g cooked chicken, skinless
    and cut into chunks

1. Preheat the oven to 180°C/160°C fan/350°F/gas mark 4.

2. Combine all the dressing ingredients – lemon juice, vinegar, olive oil and mustard – in a clean jar with a lid, shake until fully emulsified, then set aside.

3. Prepare the topping by rubbing all the ingredients together in a large bowl to a crumbly mixture with no large lumps, then set aside.

4. In a pan over a medium heat, combine the pesto and mascarpone with 250ml water. Heat and stir until smooth and bubbling, then stir in the spinach and peas. Cook until the spinach has wilted into the sauce and the peas have thawed, then add the chicken, basil, mint and a splash of milk.

5. Transfer the chicken and sauce into an ovenproof dish and cover with the crumble topping.

6. Bake for 35–40 minutes until the top is golden.

7. Pour the dressing over the lettuce and serve with the crumble.

BREAKFAST

Green mushroom and ricotta crêpes

I love pancakes; it's probably a throwback to living in America when I was small. These pancakes are packed full of vegetables, with some creaminess coming from the ricotta. Most crêpe recipes use a 1 cup of flour to 1 cup of milk to 1 egg ratio, but adding the spinach means you need a bit more milk to thin out the mixture so you are left with lovely crispy crêpes.

300 calories

50g spinach leaves
120g plain flour, sifted
240ml milk
2 eggs, whisked
Zest of 1 lemon
Pinch of pepper

1 tbsp olive oil
400g chestnut mushrooms, chopped
200g ricotta cheese
Small bunch of chives, chopped

---

1. Use a blender to chop the spinach very finely.

2. Put the spinach purée into a mixing bowl with the flour, milk, eggs, lemon zest and pepper and set aside while you make the filling.

3. In a pan over a medium heat, add the olive oil and then the mushrooms. Pan-fry for about 8 minutes, until slightly crispy and golden brown, then set aside.

4. Using the same pan, heat over a medium heat and add a tiny bit of the olive oil so the pancakes don't stick.

5. Pour about three quarters of a cup of the batter into the frying pan, rotating the pan as you do this so that the batter spreads quickly across the base. When you can see the edges of the pancake beginning to lighten in colour, it is about done on one side – this will take about 2 minutes. At this point, flip the pancake over and cook it on the other side. Repeat until all the batter is used (you should make four pancakes, but if you are using a smaller pan you may make more).

6. Spoon the ricotta, chives and mushrooms evenly into the centre of each pancake, then roll them up to serve. If you prefer, you can bring all the ingredients to the table and everyone can assemble their own.

LUNCH

One-pot roast chicken

Sunday lunch is, in my opinion, one of Britain's finest traditions. However, often Sunday lunch requires a lot of effort in cooking and washing-up, and is high in fat, so high in calories, too. This healthier version involves cooking the chicken in a pot with the veggies, so instead of using fat to cook the potatoes and veg you use the chicken juices.

750 calories

1 medium-sized chicken (approx. 1.5kg)
1 lemon, cut in half
50g unsalted butter, softened
2 garlic cloves, thinly sliced
750g new potatoes, washed and cut in half
200g carrots, peeled and chopped into chunks
200g parsnips, peeled and chopped into chunks
100g beetroot, chopped into chunks
2 tbsp olive oil
Pinch of salt and pepper
2 tsp dried oregano
200g cherry tomatoes
300g green beans, trimmed

1. Preheat the oven to 220°C/200°C fan/425°F/gas mark 7.

2. Snip the string off the chicken (if it has one holding it together) and put the lemon halves into the bird's cavity. Place the chicken in the centre of a large roasting tin and rub the skin with butter all over.

3. Cut slits about 1cm long and 1cm deep through the skin of the chicken breasts. Into each slit insert a slice of garlic.

4. Arrange the potatoes and root vegetables around the chicken. Drizzle with the olive oil, season with a pinch of salt and pepper, add the oregano and toss them all to combine thoroughly.

5. Roast the chicken for 20 minutes, then turn down the oven to 200°C/180°C fan/400°F/gas mark 6 and roast for another 50 minutes.

6. Stir the cherry tomatoes into the vegetables and return to the oven for another 10 minutes.

7. Boil the green beans for about 3 minutes, until soft.

8. Slice the chicken and serve with the roasted vegetables and green beans.

__Sunday__

DINNER

Sundried tomato and mozzarella tart with rocket and walnut pesto

This tart is incredibly easy to make and a real crowdpleaser. The traditional 'mozzarella tricolore' Italian flavours take on a new twist in this pastry dish. Although here it is a dinner recipe, it actually makes for great leftovers for lunches, too. However, as it is one of my favourite all-time recipes, I very rarely manage to have any leftovers...

540 calories

FOR THE TART
1 sheet all-butter puff pastry
    (either buy from the fridge
    section of a supermarket, or
    from frozen and thaw first)
1 x 225g jar of sundried
    tomatoes in oil, well drained
100g mozzarella, sliced
Pinch of pepper
1 egg, beaten

FOR THE WALNUT PESTO
150g rocket
1 garlic clove, peeled
150g Parmesan, grated
150g walnuts
300ml olive oil
Juice of 1 lemon

TO SERVE
150g rocket

1. Preheat the oven to 200°C/180°C fan/400°F/gas mark 6.

2. Start by making the pesto. Blitz all the ingredients together in a blender until smooth and set aside.

3. Line a baking tray with baking parchment to stop the tart sticking.

4. If the pastry comes in a block, use a rolling pin to roll the pastry out until it is about 2mm thick. If it comes ready-rolled, lay it out on the baking parchment. Using a fork, lightly prick the pastry. Next, take a knife and gently score a 2.5cm border around the edge. You don't want to accidentally cut through the pastry, but this step is essential to allow the sides of the tart to rise.

5. Arrange the sundried tomatoes and mozzarella on the pastry, making sure they stay inside the scored line. Season with the pepper.

6. Brush the edges of the pastry with the beaten egg. Bake for 20 minutes, or until golden and cooked through. Drizzle the tart with about 2 tablespoons of pesto per portion – saving the rest in a clean container in the fridge for later recipes – and serve with the rocket alongside.

Get ahead

Like many of these recipes, the breakfast for tomorrow needs some preparation the night before. However, this does mean you'll wake up tomorrow to a delicious, healthy breakfast with minimal effort.

Monday

BREAKFAST

Apricot, blueberry and hazelnut chia pudding

The combination of blueberries and hazelnuts in this recipe give it a lovely natural sweetness and a bit of 'crunch'. I love blueberries – they are full of flavour and make great snacks, too. They are often hailed as 'superfoods' – to read more about what this means, see page 266.

356 calories

500ml milk
½ tsp vanilla extract
100g dried apricots, cut into slivers
120g chia seeds

200g Greek yoghurt
50g hazelnuts, to decorate
200g blueberries (or other berries if you prefer)

1. Stir together the milk, vanilla extract, apricots and chia seeds. Refrigerate for 15 minutes then stir again. Divide among four smaller bowls, cover and refrigerate overnight.

2. In the morning, remove the chia pudding from the fridge, layer it with the Greek yoghurt and scatter over the nuts and berries, then serve.

Get ahead

Dinner this evening includes a delicious, slightly spicy, marinated lamb. I would recommend making the marinade now, pouring it over the lamb, covering it and refrigerating it until dinner. It'll make the lamb taste really delicious.

LUNCH

Peach, mozzarella and Parma ham salad

Just eating this salad makes me feel like I'm on holiday – sweet juicy peaches with creamy mozzarella and salty Parma ham is a delicious combination. Cured meats such as Parma ham are high in salt, and while you don't have to avoid all cured and processed meats completely, it is best to eat them in moderation.
Here I use just enough to give you a delicious flavour without a salt overload.

332 calories

FOR THE SALAD
250g ciabatta bread, torn into
   pieces
100g Parma ham, sliced
4 fresh peaches, stoned and
   sliced

Small handful of mint leaves,
   chopped
125g mozzarella, torn
100g rocket
Dressing from Saturday's
   dinner

1. Combine all the salad ingredients in a large bowl, tossing well to mix, then pour over some dressing and toss again.

DINNER

Harissa-marinated lamb kebabs with Greek salad

I absolutely love Middle Eastern food; I think this is predominantly because it is food made for sharing and enjoying with friends and family, and it is often packed full of vegetables. Lamb is a delicious meat, but make sure you buy good quality otherwise it can be very fatty and tough (I also buy carefully for ethical reasons, but that is up to you).

If you are using wooden skewers here, make sure you soak them in cold water for a few minutes before threading them with the meat and vegetables, to prevent them burning under the grill.

679 calories

FOR THE MARINADE
2 tbsp harissa paste
Small bunch of coriander
2 garlic cloves, peeled
Juice of ½ lime
Pinch of pepper

FOR THE KEBABS
400g lamb steak, trimmed of
   fat and chopped into chunks
2 red onions, each cut into
   eight wedges
2 red peppers, deseeded and
   chopped into large chunks

FOR THE SALAD
4 large plum tomatoes, diced
1 cucumber, diced
1 tbsp dried oregano
1 tbsp olive oil
Pinch of salt and pepper
200g pack of feta cheese
Handful of black olives
   (optional)

TO SERVE
4 wholemeal pittas, toasted

1. Turn the grill to a medium heat.

2. In a blender, blend all the marinade ingredients together until smooth.

3. Put the lamb chunks into a bowl and pour over the marinade, then set aside in the fridge for a few hours.

4. Remove the lamb chunks from the marinade and thread onto skewers, alternating them with pieces of red onion and pepper.

5. Grill for about 10 minutes, turning regularly so that they cook evenly on all sides.

6. While the lamb is cooking, make the Greek salad by combining all the ingredients.

7. To serve, assemble the Greek salad with the lamb kebab and pitta on a plate.

Tip: Although I often try to avoid cooking with salt, or use a minimal amount, in this recipe you do need a good pinch as it really helps draw the juice out of the tomatoes, and is important for flavour.

Get ahead

Dinner tomorrow is delicious, fresh-tasting marinated chicken breasts, so it's best to start the marinade the night before so the flavour really gets into the flesh of the chicken.

BREAKFAST

Menemen

Menemen are Turkish-style lightly scrambled eggs that are full of veggies. They make the perfect breakfast as they are high in protein and count towards your five-a-day.

302 calories

1 tbsp olive oil
1 red onion, diced
1 garlic clove, minced
200g cherry tomatoes, cut in half

2 red peppers, deseeded and finely chopped
4 eggs, beaten
4 slices of sourdough brown bread (from the freezer)

1. In a pan over a low–medium heat, add the olive oil then sweat down the onion and garlic. This should take about 5 minutes. Add the cherry tomatoes and peppers and cook until soft, which should take another 5 minutes.

2. Add the eggs and stir, slowly, until scrambled, for about 4 minutes.

3. Remove the eggs from the pan and pile them on top of hot toast to serve.

LUNCH

Pesto chickpea salad with cherry tomatoes

Healthy eating means different things to different people. To me, it's all about lots of fruit and vegetables and protein – both from animal and non-animal sources. This salad is so colourful and fresh, with protein from the mozzarella and chickpeas, and as it uses the pesto made earlier in the week it is very quick to put together.

440 calories

Leftover walnut pesto from
  Sunday evening
2 x 400g tins of chickpeas,
  rinsed and drained
200g cherry tomatoes, cut
  in half

Handful of black olives, pitted
  and cut in half
200g mozzarella, torn
Handful of rocket leaves
Pinch of pepper

1. Mix all the ingredients together and serve.

DINNER

Chicken skewers with rainbow slaw and warm pittas

There are very few foods I don't like, but mayonnaise is definitely one of them. So when I found a delicious dressing for a crunchy slaw that is happily mayonnaise-free, I couldn't get enough of it! This recipe is a great healthier alternative to a kebab. Still with the meat skewer and pitta, but full of fresh crunchy vegetables instead!

400 calories

FOR THE CHICKEN
1 tsp chilli flakes
Zest and juice of 2 limes
2 tbsp soy sauce
1 tsp fish sauce
1 garlic clove, minced
Salt and pepper, to taste
3 skinless chicken breasts
Olive oil, for frying

FOR THE SALAD
2 carrots, very finely sliced into
  matchsticks

2 spring onions, finely sliced
½ white cabbage, finely
  shredded
Juice of 1 lime
2 tbsp cider vinegar
2 tsp English mustard
4 tbsp olive oil

TO SERVE
4 wholemeal pittas, toasted

1. Start by making the marinade for the chicken: just combine all the ingredients except the chicken and olive oil in a medium bowl.

2. Cut the chicken breasts into chunks and add to the bowl of marinade. Cover with cling film and leave for at least 1 hour in the fridge. If you are able to do this in advance, do, as it gives the chicken the best flavour.

3. Thread the chicken onto skewers (see page 202 if you are using wooden skewers).

4. Pour the olive oil into a large frying pan (big enough to fit the kebabs) over a high heat. Cook the kebabs on all sides, starting with a high heat to get a good colour, then reducing it to cook them through; it should take about 10 minutes.

5. Meanwhile, combine all salad ingredients in a large bowl and stir thoroughly to mix.

6. Serve the chicken skewers with warm pitta and the crunchy slaw.

BREAKFAST

Porridge with rhubarb and ginger

This porridge is very quick to make, and really fresh-tasting thanks to the rhubarb and ginger. Rhubarb can be difficult to find when not in season, so I sometimes bulk-buy when I can and keep it in the freezer. If you are cooking from frozen, follow the same method below but the first step may take slightly longer.

297 calories

1 tsp unsalted butter
400g rhubarb, cut into 2cm
   pieces
Thumb-sized piece of root
   ginger, grated

150g rolled oats
750ml milk
1 tsp ground cinnamon

1. Melt the butter in a saucepan over a low heat. Add the rhubarb and ginger and cook for about 15 minutes, until very soft.

2. Add the oats, milk and cinnamon. Cook for another 5 minutes, stirring constantly, until the oats have absorbed all the milk and a creamy porridge has formed. Serve immediately.

LUNCH

Artichoke, broad bean and feta salad

Artichokes are, in my opinion, one of the most amazing vegetables. They are so full of flavour and they make a humble lunchtime salad so much more interesting!

410 calories

200g frozen broad beans
400g couscous
300g jar of artichoke hearts, drained and patted dry, then sliced

1 small bulb of fennel, very thinly sliced
1 x 200g rocket
250g feta cheese, crumbled
1 cucumber, cut into chunks

1. In a pan of water, boil the broad beans for about 3 minutes, until cooked through. Drain and allow to cool.

2. Meanwhile, prepare the couscous according to the packet instructions.

3. Mix all the other ingredients together in a bowl, add the beans and couscous, then divide among four plates.

DINNER

Smoked mackerel kedgeree

Kedgeree is thought to have originated as an Indian dish, which was then brought back to England in Victorian times by colonials, where it became popular as a breakfast dish. It's a great way to enjoy oily fish, which is good for your heart. Some versions contain cream, but this lower-calorie, lower-fat version is equally delicious and better for you.

Under 600 calories

1 tbsp olive oil
1 white onion, finely diced
2 tsp medium curry powder
300g brown rice
600ml water
3 eggs

300g cooked smoked
    mackerel fillets
Handful of parsley, finely
    chopped, to serve

1. In a large pan, heat the olive oil over a medium heat and add the onion. Fry for about 5 minutes, until soft and fragrant, before adding the spices and frying for another few minutes, until they are aromatic.

2. Add the rice to the spiced onion and stir to ensure it is well combined. Pour over the water and simmer for about 30 minutes, until all the liquid is absorbed.

3. Meanwhile, boil the eggs for about 8 minutes, until hard-boiled. Allow them to cool before peeling them and cutting them lengthways into quarters.

4. Remove the mackerel from its skin and flake. Stir the mackerel into the rice.

5. To serve, spoon the kedgeree into the middle of a plate and scatter over the hard-boiled eggs and parsley.

Get ahead

The frittata for lunch tomorrow is delicious fresh, but it also stores well in an airtight container in the fridge for a few days. If you want to take it cold to work or school in a lunchbox, making it tonight will save you time tomorrow morning.

BREAKFAST

Spicy scrambled eggs

Eggs make a great breakfast – they are quick to cook, filling, high in protein and versatile. Adding spices really adds flavour, and sprinkling eggs with coriander and spring onions at the end adds a great 'crunch', too.

273 calories

1 tsp olive oil
1 red onion, diced
1 tsp ground cumin
2 tsp paprika
Small bunch of coriander, finely chopped (leaves and stalks separated)
Pinch of chilli flakes, to taste

4 large tomatoes, cut into small chunks
4 eggs, whisked
4 slices of sourdough brown bread (from the freezer), toasted
4 spring onions, sliced

1. Heat the olive oil in a frying pan over a medium heat.

2. Add the red onion, cumin, paprika, turmeric, coriander stalks and chilli flakes. Cook for about 5 minutes, until the onion begins to soften.

3. Add the tomatoes and cook for a further 3 minutes, until they begin to soften.

4. Turn down the heat to low–medium and add the eggs. Stir continuously but gently on a low heat, until the eggs are cooked through and scrambled, 2–3 minutes.

5. Pile up your toast with the spicy scrambled eggs and sprinkle with spring onions and coriander leaves.

LUNCH

Roast vegetable and goat's cheese frittata

Frittatas make a delicious, protein-filled lunch and are great either hot (straight out of the oven) or cold, sliced in a lunchbox. They are also a good way to use up fridge leftovers – just add vegetables, soft cheese and even meat to the eggy custard base and you will create something delicious.

474 calories

1 aubergine, cut into small chunks	2 tbsp olive oil
1 courgette, cut into small chunks	200g cherry tomatoes
1 red onion, cut into eight wedges	150g hard goat's cheese, cut into small chunks
2 garlic cloves, minced	6 eggs
	300ml low-fat crème fraîche
	Pinch of pepper

1. Preheat the oven to 200°C/180°C fan/400°F/gas mark 6.

2. In a roasting dish, put the aubergine, courgette, red onion, garlic and olive oil. Toss to coat and roast for about 20 minutes.

3. Add the cherry tomatoes and roast for another 15 minutes, until all the vegetables are soft and beginning to caramelise.

4. Remove the vegetables and tip into a large deep ovenproof frying pan. Sprinkle the goat's cheese over the vegetables.

5. Whisk the eggs, crème fraîche and pepper together, then pour the egg mixture over the vegetables.

6. Cook over a low–medium heat for about 5 minutes, until the mixture is beginning to set.

7. Heat the grill, and grill the omelette for about 15 minutes, until the eggs are well set and the top of the frittata is beginning to go golden brown. Alternatively, if you don't have a grill, cook in an oven at 220°C/200°C fan/425°F/gas mark 7 for 10 minutes.

Thursday

DINNER

Asparagus and lemon pearl barley risotto

Risotto is one of my favourite comfort foods and something I make very often. Not only is it incredibly easy to make, but you can pack it full of flavour, too. This recipe, with tangy lemon and delicious roasted asparagus, is also full of texture and colour. The pearl barley gives it a slightly more 'nutty' texture and taste than standard risotto.

There is a lot of asparagus here, but you will save half of it for tomorrow's lunch.

471 calories

500g asparagus
2 tbsp olive oil
Salt and pepper, to taste
1 white onion, roughly diced
2 celery sticks
2 garlic cloves, diced

1 vegetable stock cube/stock
    pot
300g pearl barley
Zest and juice of 2 lemons
100g Parmesan, grated

1. Preheat the oven to 220°C/200°C fan/425°F/gas mark 7.

2. Snap off the tough ends of the asparagus between your
    fingers. You can do this with a knife, cutting about 2cm off
    the end of each spear, but doing it with your fingers makes
    sure you get the right breaking point and so you discard only
    the tough ends, not the soft spears.

3. In a baking dish, spread out the asparagus and drizzle with 1
    tablespoon of olive oil. Season with salt and pepper and roast
    for about 20 minutes, until soft.

4. Meanwhile, make the risotto. In a blender, chop the onion,
    celery and garlic together. Put this in a saucepan over a low-
    medium heat with the remaining olive oil and cook for a few
    minutes, until fragrant.

5. Prepare the stock, according to the packet instructions.

6. Add the pearl barley and stir to fully combine. Add one ladle
    of the stock and stir until the barley soaks up all the water.
    Continue doing this until the pearl barley has absorbed all the
    liquid, and it is soft and cooked through.

7. Remove the asparagus from the oven. Take out half of the
    spears, cover and refrigerate for tomorrow evening.

8. Remove the risotto from the hob and stir through the lemon
    zest and juice and the Parmesan. Divide among bowls and lay
    the asparagus spears on top of each. Season with pepper and
    serve immediately.

BREAKFAST

Carrot and sultana drop scones

Drop scones are like mini pancakes – they are very easy to make, and are perfect for breakfast or even cold as a delicious snack.

324 calories

200g plain flour
1 tsp baking powder
2 tsp grated nutmeg
2 large eggs
2 carrots, grated
200g plain yoghurt, plus extra

to serve (optional)
200ml milk
200g sultanas
1 tsp vegetable oil
Berries, to serve (optional)

1. Mix all the ingredients together in a medium bowl, except the vegetable oil.

2. In a pan over a medium heat, put a few drops of oil just to stop the batter sticking. Cook a few tablespoons of the batter per drop scone, cooking in batches until you have used up all the mixture. Serve hot or cold, with extra yoghurt or berries if you like.

LUNCH

Ricotta, pea and asparagus tartine

You can enjoy this tartine hot or cold – but personally I prefer it cold as it is really fresh-tasting. The combination of lemon and mint is full of flavour and as it is piled high with asparagus and peas, it actually counts for one of your five-a-day! This recipe is also delicious as a sandwich, which may make it easier to take to school or work for lunch.

332 calories

200g frozen peas
4 slices of sourdough brown
  bread (from the freezer)
200g ricotta cheese
250g asparagus (leftover from
  last night's dinner)

Zest of 1 lemon
Small handful of mint, leaves
  torn
Pepper, to taste

1. In a pan of boiling water, boil the peas for about 1 minute, until cooked through. You can boil them for longer, but personally I prefer them with a bit of 'bite'.

2. Drain the peas and put them into a small bowl. Using the back of a fork, roughly mash the peas (this will help them stay on top of the bread, otherwise they roll everywhere!).

3. Spread the sourdough slices with ricotta, then pile on the peas and asparagus, then top with lemon zest and mint. Season with pepper.

DINNER

Hake with hasselback potatoes and braised veggies

Hake is a really delicious white fish, and a good source of lean protein. However, if you struggle to find it in the shops, you can always substitute it with cod. I like this recipe because of the different textures – soft fish with crunchy potatoes is a great combination.

430 calories

FOR THE POTATOES
600g new potatoes
2 tbsp olive oil
Salt and pepper, to taste

FOR THE VEGGIES
1 tbsp olive oil
100g bacon lardons
3 celery sticks, finely chopped

1 white onion, diced
2 small carrots, diced
1 garlic clove, minced
½ white cabbage, shredded
2 tsp dried thyme
4 hake fillets
300ml vegetable stock (made
  with a stock cube)

1. Preheat the oven to 200°C/180°C fan/400°F/gas mark 6.

2. Start by preparing the potatoes. Place one potato on a wooden spoon, and starting at one end make cuts widthways three quarters of the way through the potato. The wooden spoon will stop you cutting right through. Repeat for all the potatoes. Put the potatoes into a roasting dish and drizzle with olive oil and season with salt and pepper. Roast for 45 minutes, until crispy.

3. To make the veggies, heat the olive oil in a shallow frying pan with a lid. Add the lardons, celery, onion, carrots and garlic and cook until soft, about 5 minutes. Add the cabbage and thyme, then stir well to combine. Place the hake on top of the veggies, pour over the stock and put the lid on. Turn the heat down to low and allow the fish to gently steam for 6–8 minutes, until cooked through.

4. Serve the hake on a bed of vegetables, with the potatoes alongside.

Recipes: Week 5

N.B. Each meal serves four people
unless otherwise stated.

MENU

	Breakfast	Lunch	Dinner
Saturday	Crumpet French toast with whipped ricotta and berries	Smoked chicken quesadilla	Aubergine Parmigiana
Sunday	Breakfast burritos	Rainbow vegetable tart	Mushroom, kale and Cheddar savoury oatmeal

SHOPPING LIST

Carbohydrate

☐ 8 wholemeal tortilla wraps

☐ 8 crumpets

Dairy products:

☐ 350g Cheddar

☐ 200g mozzarella

☐ 250g Parmesan

☐ 2 pints of milk

☐ 350ml crème fraîche

☐ 250g ricotta

Meat, fish and meat alternatives

☐ 2 smoked chicken breasts

☐ 8 eggs

Fruits/vegetables

☐ 2 white onions

☐ 1 red onion

☐ 1 bulb garlic

☐ 400g chestnut mushrooms

☐ 200g kale

☐ 2 aubergines

☐ 1 bunch of spring onions

☐ 3 avocados

☐ 2 red peppers

☐ 250g asparagus

☐ 500g carrots

☐ 350g mixed berries

Other – dried larder foods

☐ 2 x 400g tins of chopped tomatoes

☐ Jalapenos (optional!)

☐ 1 x 400g tin of refried beans (check the label to ensure no added sugar)

Fresh herbs

☐ Coriander

BREAKFAST

Crumpet French toast with whipped ricotta and berries

I absolutely love crumpets; to me they are the ultimate British teatime treat. But they actually lend themselves to making French toast perfectly, as they are so good at soaking up the 'eggy' mixture. Often French toast is served dripping in honey or syrup, but this is a low-sugar alternative, which I think is equally satisfying.

Under 450 calories

FOR THE FRENCH TOAST
2 eggs
300ml milk
1 tsp vanilla extract
1 tsp grated nutmeg
1 tsp ground cinnamon
8 crumpets
1 tsp unsalted butter

FOR THE WHIPPED RICOTTA
250g ricotta
2 tsp vanilla extract

TO SERVE
350g mixed berries

1. Whisk the eggs together with the milk, vanilla extract and spices. Place the crumpets in the mixture, cover and put in the fridge for 30 minutes.

2. Meanwhile, make the whipped ricotta. Combine the ricotta with the vanilla extract in a bowl, and whip until light and fluffy with a hand whisk or using an electric whisk if you have one.

3. To cook the crumpets, melt the butter in a frying pan and place the crumpets in, smooth side down. Spoon more eggy mixture over the top and cook for about 5 minutes, before flipping and repeating on the other side.

4. Remove the crumpets from the pan, and pile high with the whipped ricotta and berries, then serve.

LUNCH

Smoked chicken quesadilla

Smoked chicken makes a lovely change from normal chicken – the flavour is amazing and quite strong, so it is best used in a dish that really shows it off. This quesadilla is incredibly quick and easy to make – make it as spicy as you dare.

Makes 2 quesadillas (each tortilla serves 2 people, cut into wedges)
Under 600 calories

½ tsp olive oil
4 wholemeal tortilla wraps
2 smoked chicken breasts, cut
   into thin strips
100g Cheddar cheese, grated
Jalapenos (optional – as many
   as you dare!)

3 spring onions, sliced
2 avocados, stoned, peeled and
   sliced
Handful of coriander leaves,
   roughly chopped

1. Put a small amount of olive oil in a non-stick frying pan, and add one tortilla.

2. Pile half the chicken, Cheddar, Jalapenos (if using), spring onions and avocados on top of the tortilla, then sandwich with a second tortilla wrap. Cook for about 4 minutes, pressing down regularly with the back of a spatula, until the cheese is melted and the quesadilla is holding together.

3. Flip the quesadilla over carefully and cook for another 4 minutes on the other side.

4. Remove from the pan and cut into wedges, then sprinkle with coriander to serve. Repeat for the second quesadilla.

DINNER

Aubergine Parmigiana

Aubergine Parmigiana is a dish made by layering aubergines in a similar way to making lasagna. This is one of my go-to dishes; I cook it so often I have never actually thought to look at a recipe. It is also very easy to 'scale up' if you have a crowd. Often aubergines are cooked in lots of oil, but I think they are just as tasty roasted – not to mention much, much lower in calories!

500 calories

2 aubergines	2 tsp balsamic vinegar
2 tbsp olive oil	200g mozzarella, sliced
Salt and pepper	100g Parmesan
2 garlic cloves, minced	100g breadcrumbs, or 2 slices
1 white onion, diced	of bread, grated
1 tbsp dried oregano	
2 x 400g tins of chopped	
tomatoes	

1. Slice the aubergines thinly, sprinkle with half the olive oil, season with salt and pepper, and arrange them on a baking tray – it doesn't matter if they overlap slightly. Roast for 15 minutes, until soft and slightly golden brown.

2. Meanwhile, in a pan over a medium heat, fry the garlic and onion in the remaining olive oil, until aromatic. Add the oregano and stir well to combine.

3. Add the chopped tomatoes and balsamic vinegar, then allow the mixture to simmer for about 20 minutes to allow the flavours to develop.

4. Preheat the oven to 220°C/200°C fan/425°F/gas mark 7.

5. Pour a little of the tomato mixture into a rectangular baking dish to cover the base. Layer some aubergine slices on top, then some mozzarella and pour over enough tomato sauce to cover. Repeat this until all the tomato mixture, aubergines and mozzarella are used up, finishing with a layer of tomato sauce.

6. Sprinkle the Parmesan and breadcrumbs on the top, then bake for 30 minutes, until bubbling and the top is golden brown.

BREAKFAST

Breakfast burritos

I love Mexican food – I think it comes from living in America when I was little where Mexican food was everywhere, and so fresh and delicious. Often burritos are thought of as a dinner food, but they make a fantastic breakfast, too.

About 550 calories

FOR THE VEGGIE BEAN MIX

1 tsp olive oil

1 garlic clove, minced

1 red onion, cut into eight half-moons

2 red peppers, deseeded and cut into strips

Pinch of chilli flakes, to taste

1 tsp ground cumin

1 tsp paprika

1 x 400g tin of refried beans (check the label to make sure they have no added sugar!)

TO SERVE

4 wholemeal flour tortillas

1 avocado, stoned and cut into strips

2 spring onions, chopped

Small bunch of coriander, chopped

100g Cheddar cheese, grated

50ml crème fraîche

1. In a pan over a medium heat, add the olive oil, garlic, red onion and red peppers, and cook for about 5 minutes, until soft. Add the spices and stir to combine. Add the refried beans and cook for another few minutes, until well cooked through and hot.

2. Warm the tortillas according to the packet instructions.

3. To serve, divide the veggie bean mix among the four tortillas, placing the mix in the centre. Pile with the avocado, spring onions, coriander, cheddar and crème fraîche. Fold one side of the tortilla wrap in, then the opposite side. These will form the 'ends' that will stop the contents spilling out. Fold over the final two sides and enjoy.

LUNCH

Rainbow vegetable tart

This is without a doubt the prettiest recipe in the book. By layering vegetables that alternate in colour you get beautiful slices of tart. However, make sure that when you slice the tart you do this carefully – you don't want to break up the layers. I find a serrated knife is useful here.

Under 500 calories

250g frozen broad beans
500g carrots, peeled and cut into batons
250g asparagus, about 2.5cm cut off the ends

6 eggs
300ml low-fat crème fraîche
150g Parmesan, finely grated
Pepper, to taste

1. Preheat the oven to 180°C/160°C fan/350°F/gas mark 4.

2. Line an 22cm springform tin (these are usually cake tins, and I like mine with cake tin liners as it is easier than using baking parchment).

3. Cook the broad beans in boiling water for 2 minutes, drain, blanch in cold water and place in the bottom of the tin.

4. Boil the carrots for 3 minutes so the batons are still slightly crunchy, then drain, blanch in cold water and scatter over the broad beans.

5. Boil the asparagus for 2 minutes, drain, blanch in cold water and place on top of the carrots.

6. Whisk the eggs, crème fraîche, Parmesan and pepper together.

7. Pour the eggy custard mix over the layered vegetables and bake for 35 minutes, until the egg mixture is set.

8. Allow the tart to cool before slicing – this will make sure it keeps its shape.

DINNER

Mushroom, kale and Cheddar savoury oatmeal

Often people think porridge is only a breakfast food, sweetened with syrups and fruit. However, traditionally it was made with salt and water. This recipe takes porridge back to its roots, but with a modern (and tastier) twist. Porridge oats are a great source of soluble fibre, which is good for your heart.

525 calories

240g rolled oats
500ml milk
1 tsp salt
200g kale, stalks removed
1 tbsp olive oil
1 medium white onion, diced

2 garlic cloves, minced
400g chestnut mushrooms
2 tsp dried thyme
Pepper, to taste
150g Cheddar, grated

1. In a pan over a low heat, combine the oats, milk, salt and kale and cook for 15–20 minutes, so that the oats absorb all the moisture. Do this nice and slowly so that the oats become creamier.

2. In a saucepan over a medium heat, heat the olive oil then add the onion and garlic. Sauté for about 3 minutes, until they begin to soften. Add the mushrooms and thyme and cook until the mushrooms are golden brown and slightly crispy on the outside.

3. Serve the crispy mushrooms in bowls topped with the creamy oatmeal, lots of pepper and the grated Cheddar.

Snacks

Rocket, prosciutto and Parmesan frittata bites

These are incredibly easy to make and delicious. They really rise in the oven and look very pretty, so if you can, eat them whilst they are still hot. They will keep in the fridge in a sealed container for a few days, so you can always have them as an on-the-go snack, too. The balance of egg, cheese and a small amount of meat means they are high in protein, which is great for keeping you full all morning.

Makes 8 bites
Under 100 calories

4 slices of prosciutto, cut in
   half each
Handful of rocket
3 eggs

2 tbsp crème fraîche
Pinch of salt and pepper
50g grated Parmesan

1. Preheat the oven to 200°C/180°C fan/400°F/gas mark 6.

2. Arrange half a slice of prosciutto and a small amount of rocket in each well of the muffin tin.

3. Whisk together the eggs, crème fraîche, salt, pepper and Parmesan.

4. Pour the egg mixture over the prosciutto and rocket.

5. Bake for 20 minutes, until the frittata bites have puffed up and are golden brown on top.

Banana and coconut fro-yo

When people go sugar-free they often miss desserts – and ice cream is frequently top of the list. This far healthier alternative uses a blended frozen banana, so it even counts as one of your five-a-day.

Serves 4
Under 300 calories per portion

2 bananas, frozen
500g coconut-milk yoghurt

2 tsp vanilla extract

1. Blend all the ingredients together in a food processor, until completely smooth. Part way through, you may need to scrape down the side of the bowl to make sure there are no lumps left.

2. You can eat this now, but it won't be completely solid, so it's best to transfer it to an airtight freezable container and freeze for a further few hours. Use within 1 month.

Pitta fingers with tzatziki

The addition of pomegranate seeds and pistachio nuts takes the tzatziki to the next level – you get crunch from the nuts, sweet bursts of juiciness from the pomegranate and punch from the garlic.

Serves 4
Under 300 calories per portion

FOR THE TZATZIKI

½ cucumber
170g Greek yoghurt
Small handful of mint leaves
1 garlic clove, minced
Juice of ½ lemon
2 tsp olive oil

Pinch of salt and pepper
100g pomegranate seeds
50g pistachio nuts (optional)

TO SERVE

4 wholemeal pitta breads,
    toasted and cut into fingers

---

1. First make the tzatziki. Start by grating the cucumber, then wrap it in kitchen paper and press down to drain some of the water. Put it in a mixing bowl with all other tzatziki ingredients and mix well to combine.

2. Serve with toasted pitta bread fingers.

Spicy baked plantain chips

A great alternative to crisps, these are baked rather than fried, so they are lower in fat (and therefore calories). Plantain is also a great source of fibre and several vitamins and minerals, including vitamins A, B6 and C, and potassium. Either serve warm or keep in an airtight container to snack on at home or at work over the next few days.

Serves 2
100 calories per portion

1 green plantain (don't worry if it has black spots on the skin – this won't affect the flesh)

1 tbsp olive oil
Salt and pepper, to taste
Pinch of chilli flakes

1. Preheat the oven to 200°C/180°C fan/400°F/gas mark 6.

2. Use a sharp knife to peel the plantain, before slicing it as thinly as possible. If you have a mandolin, this may help, but if not, just take your time.

3. In a bowl, combine the plantain, olive oil, salt, pepper and chilli flakes. Use your hands to mix, so that the plantain slices are well coated.

4. Cover a baking tray with baking parchment, then lay out the plantain slices, ensuring they do not overlap.

5. Bake in the oven for 8–10 minutes per side, until crispy. When they are cooked, they will start to brown around the edges.

Snacks

Green medley of crudités with a tahini dip

The crunchy crudités here perfectly complement the tahini dip. Mix up the crudités to suit your tastes (and use up what you have in the fridge!). How about carrots or orange peppers for a vibrant orange version?

Serves 4
200 calories per portion

180g cream cheese
2 tbsp tahini
Juice of 1 lemon
2 tsp harissa paste

½ head of broccoli, broken into small florets
2 celery sticks, cut into sticks
½ cucumber, cut into sticks

1. Blend the cream cheese, tahini, lemon and harissa paste together.

2. Serve with the vegetables as dips.

Snacks

Pitta fingers with a beetroot dip

This snack is sure to impress people – the colour is so vibrant and the taste is amazing, owing to the 'zing' from the horseradish.

Serves 4
300 calories per portion

2 beetroots
Juice of 1 lemon
Generous handful of parsley
3 garlic cloves, peeled
250g tinned chickpeas, rinsed
and drained
1 tbsp tahini
1 tsp horseradish
4 slices of wholemeal pitta,
toasted and cut into fingers

1. Preheat the oven to 180°C/160°C fan/350°F/gas mark 4.

2. Wrap the beetroot in tin foil and roast in the oven, until soft (about 1 hour).

3. Remove the beetroot, unwrap and leave to cool before peeling off the skin. If there are pieces of skin that are soft and difficult to remove, you can leave them on.

4. Add the beetroot flesh, lemon juice, parsley, garlic, chickpeas, tahini and horseradish to a blender, and pulse until smooth. You may need to wipe down the sides of the blender with a spatula a few times during the blending.

5. Serve with the warm pitta bread fingers.

Sourdough fingers with a creamy sundried tomato dip

The crunchiness of these sourdough fingers goes really well with the creaminess of the dip. The cream cheese adds extra protein to help keep you full.

Serves 6
Under 300 calories per portion

1 garlic bulb
1 x 180g tub of cream cheese
100g sundried tomatoes (if you bought ones in oil, drain them)

Small handful of basil
3 slices of sourdough bread, toasted and cut into fingers

1. Preheat the oven to 200°C/180°C fan/400°F/gas mark 6.

2. Begin by roasting the garlic; put the garlic bulb on a roasting tray in the oven for 40 minutes.

3. Once the garlic is done, squeeze out the garlic flesh into a blender with the remaining ingredients. Blend until smooth.

4. Serve with toasted sourdough fingers.

Sweet potato wedges with a harissa and feta dip

Sweet potatoes are a real comfort food for me. A source of carbohydrate, they are also high in fibre – particularly if you leave the skin on, as I have here.

Serves 4
150 calories per portion

2 sweet potatoes (or one very large one), cut into wedges	1 tbsp harissa
1 tsp olive oil	Zest of 1 lime
Salt and pepper, to taste	Juice of ½ lime
2 tbsp crème fraîche	100g feta, crumbled

1. Preheat the oven to 200°C/180°C fan/400°F/gas mark 6.

2. Toss the wedges in the olive oil, salt and pepper, then spread out on a baking tray.

3. Roast in the oven for 20 minutes, until lightly browned and soft through – poke them with a knife and it should pass through easily.

4. To make the dip, mix the crème fraîche, harissa, lime zest, lime juice and feta together. Serve the warm wedges with the dip.

Smoky paprika popcorn

Popcorn is a real family favourite. Usually associated with going to the movies, it is often an oily, sweet or salty treat. But it doesn't need to be – this version is full of flavour but much better for you.

Under 100 calories per portion
Serves 2

4 tbsp popping corn
1 tsp smoked paprika

1. Put the corn kernels into a non-stick saucepan over a medium heat.

2. Put a lid on top, and let the corn pop until it stops – this will take a few minutes, and you will probably have a few unpopped kernels left.

3. Remove from the heat, but while still hot shake the paprika to cover the popcorn.

Smoked mackerel pâté with homemade tortilla chips

This recipe really couldn't be easier – or more delicious. Smoked mackerel is a great way to get in some extra heart-healthy oily fish into your diet, and it's cheap, too. The addition of lemon, parsley, horseradish and Dijon mustard really brings out the flavour of the mackerel.

Serves 4
Approx. 350 calories per portion

FOR THE PÂTÉ
200g smoked mackerel fillets
200g creme fraiche
Large handful of parsley
1 tsp horseradish (more if you
  like it spicy!)
1 tsp dijon mustard
1 lemon – juice and zest

Black pepper, to taste

FOR THE TORTILLA CHIPS
4 flour tortillas (alternatively,
  you can use plain corn tortilla
  chips instead of making
  your own)

1. First, prepare the tortilla chips. Preheat the oven to 180°C/160°C fan/350°F/gas mark 4.

2. Cut the tortillas into eight, then spread them out on a baking tray, lined with non-stick paper, and bake for 6 minutes.

3. Next, make the pâté. Remove the skin from the mackerel and discard. Transfer to a blender with all the other pâté ingredients and blend until well mixed.

4. Transfer the pate to a bowl, remove the tortilla chips from the oven onto a plate, and serve.

Extra
Information

FAQs about healthy eating

SHOULD I AVOID DAIRY AND WHEAT IF I WANT TO HAVE A HEALTHY DIET?

Absolutely not. This is a common misconception; dairy is a good source of calcium and protein, and wheat is a good source of calories, which can also be high in calcium and iron – this is because, by law, flour has added calcium and often has added iron, too. Some people have lactose intolerance or cow's milk protein allergy, while others suffer from coeliac disease or non-coeliac gluten sensitivity, and if you have either or both of these conditions you will need to avoid certain foods. However, if neither of these foods cause you problems, you should not make dietary exclusions that you don't need to. In fact, a recent study found no evidence to suggest that avoiding wheat (unless you are coeliac) improves health. Furthermore, many packaged 'free-from' foods are high in unhealthy fat and sugar, so are best consumed in moderation or avoided.

You must always seek advice from a doctor or dietitian before making exclusions, as it could cause you to miss out on essential nutrients.

SHOULD I AVOID EATING CARBOHYDRATES IN THE EVENING IF I WANT TO MAINTAIN A HEALTHY WEIGHT?

Lots of people give up eating carbs in the evening (6pm is a popular cut-off), and some do lose weight by doing so. Is this because 6pm until morning are carb witching hours? Of course not. Your body will recognise carbohydrates in the same way irrespective of what time of day it is. It is the total amount of carbs that you eat throughout the day, and not the time of day at which you eat them, that is important. When people lose weight by giving up carbohydrates in the evening, it is most likely to be because they are consuming fewer calories over the course of the whole day.

HOW DO I SPOT A MISLEADING NUTRITION STUDY IN THE MEDIA?

Nutrition is a science, and as such it is constantly changing as new things are being found out about how our bodies work. So often people say to me that the ever-changing guidelines or messages are confusing, but actually they should show you that our understanding of nutrition is moving on.

However, as with all science, there are lots of grey areas, which is why, in the Facts vs Myths section, I often say 'It's complicated'. Why? Because it is! Nutrition is always in the media, so it is really important to be able to understand if a study is being well reported, because a large amount of the time it isn't.

There are a few ways you can protect yourself from 'nutritional nonsense':

1. Does it sound too good to be true? If so, it probably is.
2. Look at the credentials of the person reporting – are they a doctor, dietitian or Association for Nutrition registered nutritionist? (That's the gold standard for scientifically accurate nutrition information.) If the person making the claim is a celebrity, bear in mind that they probably do not have the scientific training to support it and that they look fabulous because they have a great make-up artist and hair stylist!
3. Look for the study they are taking about; if it is in a newspaper, you will hopefully be able to find out where the headline came from.
4. Watch out for words like 'breakthrough', 'causes' or 'proves'. These words pull in readers but often signify that the science is being over-simplified – sometimes to the point at which it is no longer true.

IS ORGANIC FOOD HEALTHIER?

The organic label can be applied when the food has been produced without the use of artificial chemicals, such as pesticides or fertilisers. Lots of people choose to buy organic because of the food's perceived nutritional or environmental benefits. This has been a booming area of scientific research, but actually (and surprisingly to most people!) studies have found very little difference in nutritional composition between organically and non-organically produced food. If you choose to buy organic food for the environmental benefits, by all means continue to do so (I buy organic when I can for this reason!), but if you are spending your money thinking that an organic cucumber is healthier than its non-organic counterpart, think again.

SHOULD I GO ON A 'DETOX' DIET?

A detox diet is one that claims to help your body rid itself of unwanted substances called toxins. Detox diets tend to be highly restrictive, and often promote specific detox products, which can be very expensive. Sometimes people feel better after doing a detox, but this is usually because they are not over-eating and because they are drinking lots of water, not smoking and are avoiding alcohol.

Our bodies are clever – one of the main functions of our liver and kidneys is to rid our bodies of waste products. Therefore, if your liver and kidneys are working well, your body is capable of doing all the detoxing that it needs. In fact, every time you go to the loo you are detoxing, as you are getting rid of waste from the body! If you feel run down, make sure you get a good night's sleep, drink lots of water, reduce your consumption of processed (fast) food, eat lots of vegetables and cut down on smoking and drinking alcohol. That's all the detoxing your body needs.
If you have a problem with your liver or kidneys, you must seek medical advice rather than try a 'detox' diet yourself.

WHAT ARE SUPERFOODS AND SHOULD I EAT THEM?

Superfoods are foods that are high in certain specific nutrients and are often hailed as the magic cure to your health, because they give you more energy and/or prevent or cure disease. However, a superfood is just a marketing term – there is nothing scientific behind these claims. This can make the word confusing – you can easily get sucked into the 'superfood' marketing world and spend lots of money on ingredients that are no better for you than any others. For example, pink Himalayan sea salt is often called a superfood for its high magnesium content, but to reach your daily requirement of magnesium you would need to eat 2kg per day of the stuff – and that much salt would be detrimental to your body. If you can afford superfoods and you want to include them in your diet, go ahead and do so in moderation, but you don't need expensive, trendy foods in your diet to be healthy. Hopefully the recipes in this book will show you that!

IS COCONUT OIL GOOD FOR ME?

Coconut oil has had a lot of good press lately for its perceived health benefits. We are in such a craze about this ingredient that, according to the UN's Food and Agriculture Organization (FAO), global demand for it is growing at 10 per cent per year and the global market for coconut water hit $2.26 billion in 2016.

It seems our appetite for coconuts is insatiable. But why? Coconut is a plant fat, and so many assumed it was good for us. However, coconut oil is about 86 per cent saturated (bad) fat, which is even higher than butter! For a while, some people thought that the fat in coconut oil was better for us than other saturated fats, but so far we don't have a good science-based answer for that. It is very likely that the saturated fats in coconuts are used in the same way by our bodies as the saturated fats in butter. But we do know that replacing saturated fats with unsaturated (good) fats is an effective way to reduce bad cholesterol levels as well as lower the risk of heart disease and stroke.

So, for now, if you like a little bit of coconut oil, use it as you would have used butter, but don't go spreading it on everything thinking you're doing your heart a favour, because the likelihood is you'll be doing the opposite! Opt instead for nuts, seeds, nut butters and other vegetable oils to provide you with the fat you need in your diet. The recipes in this book focus highly on olive oils and nuts instead of butter and high-fat dairy for just this reason.

ARE EGGS BAD FOR ME?

Eggs are a great source of protein, as well as many vitamins and minerals – including vitamins D, A, B2 and B12, folate and iodine. However, there is a common belief that eggs cause us to have a high cholesterol (a high level of fat in our blood, which can lead to increased risk of heart attacks and strokes) and therefore we should eat a maximum of two per week. This is, in fact, a misconception – although eggs contain cholesterol, the amount of saturated fat (unhealthy fat) we eat has more of an effect on the cholesterol in our blood than the cholesterol we get from food such as eggs. If you have high cholesterol, you will need to be careful about your saturated fat intake, and it is worth speaking to a doctor or dietitian about how to go about this.

There is no upper limit on the number of eggs you can eat, and they make a good contribution to a healthy diet, as well as being quick to cook and cheap, too.

Index

Recipe Index

Acknowledgements

Firstly, thank you to all those people who have taught me to cook... My mother deserves a special mention – her endless patience when I created huge amounts of mess in the kitchen from a young age has not gone unnoticed.

Secondly, to my friends who, when asking about whether 'sugar was the devil', unwittingly gave me the inspiration to write this book. They have been patient recipe testers and given me some useful ideas for the introduction for this book. Particular thanks to Isobel Steane, who as a friend and colleague has given me much support through the long days and evenings of writing and looming deadlines. You kept me sane.

Thirdly, to my patients, who inspired the FAQs and 'Fact vs Myth' sections – every question you ask is important, and we can both learn from them.

Next, to everyone who made this book a reality. Emily Barrett, my good friend and editor, for your excellent eye for detail and constant encouragement. Also to Helen Ewing, Debbie Holmes, Vincent Whiteman and Laurie Perry for brilliant design, photography and food styling.

And finally, to you! If you have devoured the recipes, learned something from the introduction or enjoyed flipping through the photographs, please get in touch. I'd love to hear all your stories and I hope that my cooking has shown you that healthy food is cheap to buy, easy to cook and delicious to eat.

About the author

Catherine Kidd is a chef, foodie and dietitian. She has always loved cooking and eating, bringing together family and friends around a dinner table to share food. She combines this with her interest in health and wellbeing, working both privately and for the NHS as a dietitian. She studied at King's College, University of London, where she received a national award for her dissertation looking at heart health and diet. *30 Days of Sugar-Free* is her second book, following on from *30 Days of Vegan*.

To contact Catherine:
Facebook: Catherine Kidd Nutrition
Instagram: catherinekiddnutrition
Twitter: CatherineKiddRD
Website: www.catherinekiddnutrition.com

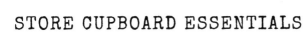

STORE CUPBOARD ESSENTIALS

Oils, vinegars and sauces

- [ ] Olive oil
- [ ] Vegetable oil
- [ ] Cider vinegar
- [ ] Balsamic vinegar
- [ ] Sesame oil
- [ ] Worcestershire sauce
- [ ] Soy sauce
- [ ] Fish sauce

Carbohydrate staples

- [ ] Plain flour
- [ ] Rolled oats
- [ ] Quinoa
- [ ] New potatoes
- [ ] Dried breadcrumbs
- [ ] Wholewheat pasta
- [ ] Brown rice
- [ ] Risotto rice
- [ ] White rice
- [ ] Wholemeal sourdough bread, sliced (or other bread, if you prefer)

Herbs, spices and flavourings

- [ ] Salt
- [ ] Pepper
- [ ] Tomato purée
- [ ] English mustard
- [ ] Tamarind paste
- [ ] Harissa paste
- [ ] Tahini
- [ ] Sriracha
- [ ] Horseradish sauce
- [ ] Vegetable stock cubes/ stock pots
- [ ] Preserved lemons
- [ ] Chilli flakes
- [ ] Dried oregano
- [ ] Mixed dried herbs
- [ ] Ground cumin
- [ ] Grated nutmeg
- [ ] Fennel seeds
- [ ] Cardamom pods
- [ ] Ground cinnamon
- [ ] Dried thyme

- [ ] Paprika
- [ ] Dried fenugreek leaves
- [ ] Ground ginger
- [ ] Mustard seeds
- [ ] Cumin seeds
- [ ] Curry powder

For the freezer

- [ ] Peas
- [ ] Broad beans
- [ ] Ice cubes/ice-cube trays
- [ ] Sliced brown bread (I like sourdough!)

For the fridge

- [ ] Unsalted butter

Other

- [ ] Bicarbonate of soda
- [ ] Baking powder
- [ ] Chia seeds
- [ ] Vanilla extract
- [ ] Capers
- [ ] Cornichons

Equipment

- [ ] Muffin tin
- [ ] Loaf tin (approx. 450g)
- [ ] Steamer

SHOPPING LIST WEEK 1

Carbohydrate

- [ ] Large olive ciabatta (from the bakery section of most supermarkets)
- [ ] 4 wholemeal burger buns
- [ ] 4 brioche buns
- [ ] 1 baguette
- [ ] 1 pack (500g) ready-made puff pastry
- [ ] 3 large baking potatoes (e.g. Maris Piper)
- [ ] 250g packet of ready-cooked Puy lentils
- [ ] 500g new potatoes

Dairy products:

- [ ] 500g Greek yoghurt
- [ ] 400ml crème fraîche
- [ ] 2 x 200g feta cheese
- [ ] 250g cream cheese
- [ ] 1 x 150g ball mozzarella
- [ ] 225g block of halloumi
- [ ] 4 pints of milk

Meat, fish and meat alternatives

- [ ] 500g turkey mince
- [ ] 400g skirt/bavette steak
- [ ] 2 pork necks
- [ ] 4 skin-on salmon fillets
- [ ] 300g Quorn mince (found in the freezer section of supermarket)
- [ ] 2 skinless chicken breasts
- [ ] 200g pack smoked mackerel
- [ ] 200g rashers of unsmoked back bacon
- [ ] 400g cod goujons
- [ ] 13 eggs

Fruits/vegetables

- [ ] 200g kale
- [ ] 2 iceberg lettuces
- [ ] 6 lemons
- [ ] 1 bulb garlic
- [ ] 4 red onions
- [ ] 3 cucumbers

- [ ] 150g watercress
- [ ] 1 white onion
- [ ] 1 head of broccoli
- [ ] 5 carrots
- [ ] 500g spinach
- [ ] 1 bunch of spring onions
- [ ] 3 bananas
- [ ] 120g rocket
- [ ] 2 Braeburn apples
- [ ] 4 plums
- [ ] 230g strawberries
- [ ] 100g green beans
- [ ] 6 medium tomatoes
- [ ] 1 mango
- [ ] 1 avocado
- [ ] 300g chestnut mushrooms

Other – dried larder foods

- [ ] 280g jar of artichoke hearts
- [ ] 1 x 400g tin of red kidney beans
- [ ] 200g cocoa nibs

- [ ] 1 x 198g tin of sweetcorn
- [ ] 1 x 400g tin of black beans

Fresh herbs

- [ ] Mint
- [ ] Coriander
- [ ] Parsley
- [ ] Dill
- [ ] Basil
- [ ] Chives

Dried fruits and nuts

- [ ] 200g prunes
- [ ] 100g raw cashews
- [ ] 250g pistachios (200g to be used in Week 4)
- [ ] 600g sultanas (200g to be used in Weeks 3 and 4)
- [ ] 280g tub of peanut butter
- [ ] 100g Medjool dates
- [ ] 100g pecans

SHOPPING LIST WEEK 2

Carbohydrate

- [ ] 4 chapatis
- [ ] 8 hard-shell tacos
- [ ] 4 wholemeal burger buns
- [ ] 220g bulgar wheat
- [ ] 4 wholewheat tortilla wraps
- [ ] Sliced rye bread
- [ ] 1 x 250g packet of ready-cooked Puy lentils

Dairy products:

- [ ] 450g feta cheese
- [ ] 2 small goat's cheese rounds
- [ ] 150g soft cheese with garlic
- [ ] 100g soured cream
- [ ] 250g Cheddar
- [ ] 250g Greek yoghurt
- [ ] 2 pints of milk
- [ ] 1 x 250g block of halloumi

Meat, fish and meat alternatives

- [ ] 3 skinless chicken breasts
- [ ] 400g good-quality pork mince
- [ ] 4 salmon fillets (approx. 500g)
- [ ] 400g frozen prawns
- [ ] 200g chorizo
- [ ] 8 chicken thighs, with skin on
- [ ] 1 litre good-quality chicken stock
- [ ] 8 rashers of unsmoked back bacon
- [ ] 12 eggs (this will give you some leftovers for next week!)

Fruits/vegetables

- [ ] 6 red onions
- [ ] 3 white onions
- [ ] 2 bulbs garlic
- [ ] 3 limes
- [ ] 300g rocket

- [ ] 9 lemons
- [ ] 4 aubergines
- [ ] 7 avocados
- [ ] 6 tomatoes
- [ ] 8 sweet potatoes
- [ ] 300g green beans
- [ ] 4 courgettes
- [ ] 3 peppers (red, orange, yellow or green – according to personal preference)
- [ ] 500g kale, large stems removed
- [ ] 500g cherry tomatoes
- [ ] 3 apples
- [ ] 400g frozen blackberries (fresh is fine – just normally more expensive)
- [ ] 200g pomegranate seeds
- [ ] 200g raspberries
- [ ] 4 bananas

Other – dried larder foods

- [ ] 2 x 400g tins of chickpeas
- [ ] 4 × 400g tins of chopped tomatoes
- [ ] 1 × 400g tin of coconut milk
- [ ] 1 x 350g can of green olives
- [ ] 1 x 330g tin of sweetcorn
- [ ] 1.5 litres hazelnut milk
- [ ] 2 x 400g tins of butter beans

Fresh herbs:

- [ ] Root ginger
- [ ] Coriander
- [ ] Parsley
- [ ] Tarragon
- [ ] Basil
- [ ] Mint

Dried fruits and nuts:

- [ ] 100g hazelnuts (use 50g in Week 4)
- [ ] 300g flaked almonds (use 50g in Week 3)
- [ ] 100g sesame seeds
- [ ] 150g cocoa nibs

SHOPPING LIST WEEK 3

Carbohydrate

- [ ] 1.5kg waxy potatoes
- [ ] 4 wholemeal pitta breads
- [ ] 300g dried rice noodles
- [ ] 4 wholemeal wraps
- [ ] 4 plain bagels
- [ ] 4 flatbreads
- [ ] 2 sweet potatoes
- [ ] 4 wholemeal bread rolls

Dairy products

- [ ] 300ml 0% fat natural yoghurt
- [ ] 1 x 250g block of halloumi
- [ ] 600g Greek yoghurt
- [ ] 300ml low-fat crème fraîche
- [ ] 550g feta cheese
- [ ] 1 x 280g tub of cream cheese
- [ ] 300g soft goat's cheese
- [ ] 3 pints of milk

Meat, fish and meat alternatives

- [ ] 300g chorizo
- [ ] 10 skinless chicken breasts
- [ ] 600g beef stewing steak
- [ ] 300g lean beef mince
- [ ] 300ml fresh beef stock
- [ ] 4 sea bass fillets
- [ ] 4 tuna steaks
- [ ] 18 eggs

Fruits/vegetables

- [ ] 1 banana
- [ ] 3 red onions
- [ ] 1 bulb garlic
- [ ] 2 large eating apples
- [ ] 200g baby spinach leaves
- [ ] 400g frozen mango chunks
- [ ] 500g strawberries (fresh or frozen)
- [ ] 2 red peppers
- [ ] 1 carrot

- ☐ 4 white onions
- ☐ 4 romaine lettuces
- ☐ 9 limes
- ☐ 1 bunch of spring onions
- ☐ 350g mangetout
- ☐ 400g tenderstem broccoli
- ☐ 2 lemons
- ☐ 100g rocket
- ☐ 2 beetroots
- ☐ 2 avocados
- ☐ 2 cucumbers
- ☐ 2 heads of pak choi
- ☐ 550g cherry tomatoes

Other – dried larder foods

- ☐ 2 x 400g tins of chopped tomatoes
- ☐ Massaman curry paste
- ☐ 2 x 400ml tins of coconut milk
- ☐ 1 x 400g tin of ready-cooked Puy lentils
- ☐ 1 x 250g packet of ready-cooked Puy lentils
- ☐ 300g red split lentils

Fresh herbs:

- ☐ Root ginger
- ☐ Coriander
- ☐ Mint
- ☐ Dill
- ☐ Parsley
- ☐ 2 lemongrass stalks

Dried fruits and nuts:

- ☐ 150g flame raisins
- ☐ 200g sultanas
- ☐ 100g dried apricots
- ☐ 150g linseeds
- ☐ 100g dessicated coconut
- ☐ 50g flaked almonds
- ☐ 250g unsalted peanuts
- ☐ 100g coconut flakes

SHOPPING LIST WEEK 4

Carbohydrate
- [ ] 250g ciabatta bread
- [ ] 8 wholemeal pittas
- [ ] 1 sheet all-butter puff pastry
- [ ] 300g pearl barley
- [ ] 400g couscous

Dairy products
- [ ] 400ml buttermilk
- [ ] 400g ricotta cheese
- [ ] 425g mozzarella
- [ ] 300g Parmesan cheese
- [ ] 3 pints of milk
- [ ] 250g tub of mascarpone
- [ ] 450g feta cheese
- [ ] 300ml low-fat crème fraîche
- [ ] 150g hard goat's cheese
- [ ] 200g Greek yoghurt
- [ ] 200g plain yoghurt

Meat, fish and meat alternatives
- [ ] 5 skinless chicken breasts
- [ ] 200g cooked prawns
- [ ] 1.4 litres fresh chicken stock
- [ ] 100g Parma ham
- [ ] 300g cooked chicken, skinless
- [ ] 1 medium-sized chicken (approx. 1.5kg)
- [ ] 300g smoked mackerel fillets
- [ ] 400g lamb steak
- [ ] 4 hake fillets
- [ ] 100g bacon lardons
- [ ] 22 eggs

Fruits/vegetables
- [ ] 400g spinach leaves
- [ ] 7 lemons
- [ ] 400g chestnut mushrooms
- [ ] 6 limes
- [ ] 4 fresh peaches
- [ ] 600g rocket
- [ ] 1 romaine lettuce
- [ ] 1 bulb garlic
- [ ] 9 carrots
- [ ] Bunch of spring onions

- [ ] 1 white cabbage
- [ ] 200g parsnips
- [ ] 100g beetroot
- [ ] 800g cherry tomatoes
- [ ] 3 white onions
- [ ] 500g asparagus
- [ ] 1 fennel bulb
- [ ] 7 celery sticks
- [ ] 4 red peppers
- [ ] 5 red onions
- [ ] 8 large plum tomatoes
- [ ] 2 cucumbers
- [ ] 1 aubergine
- [ ] 1 courgette
- [ ] 3 red chillies
- [ ] 400g rhubarb
- [ ] 200g blueberries
- [ ] 300g green beans
- [ ] Small punnet of berries (optional)

Other – dried larder foods

- [ ] 190g jar of green pesto
- [ ] 1 x 225g jar of sundried tomatoes
- [ ] Small jar of black olives
- [ ] 2 x 400g tins of chickpeas
- [ ] 300g jar of artichoke hearts
- [ ] 10g dried yeast

Fresh herbs

- [ ] Chives
- [ ] Coriander
- [ ] Ginger
- [ ] Mint
- [ ] Basil
- [ ] Parsley
- [ ] 1 lemongrass stalk
- [ ] 3 kaffir lime leaves
- [ ] Root ginger

Dried fruits and nuts

- [ ] 200g sultanas
- [ ] 200g dried cranberries
- [ ] 100g dried apricots
- [ ] 150g walnuts
- [ ] 200g pistachios
- [ ] 50g hazelnuts

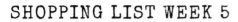

SHOPPING LIST WEEK 5

Carbohydrate

☐ 8 wholemeal tortilla wraps

☐ 8 crumpets

Dairy products:

☐ 350g Cheddar

☐ 200g mozzarella

☐ 250g Parmesan

☐ 2 pints of milk

☐ 350ml crème fraîche

☐ 250g ricotta

Meat, fish and meat alternatives

☐ 2 smoked chicken breasts

☐ 8 eggs

Fruits/vegetables

☐ 2 white onions

☐ 1 red onion

☐ 1 bulb garlic

☐ 400g chestnut mushrooms

☐ 200g kale

☐ 2 aubergines

☐ 1 bunch of spring onions

☐ 3 avocados

☐ 2 red peppers

☐ 250g asparagus

☐ 500g carrots

☐ 350g mixed berries

Other – dried larder foods

☐ 2 x 400g tins of chopped tomatoes

☐ Jalapenos (optional!)

☐ 1 x 400g tin of refried beans (check the label to ensure no added sugar)

Fresh herbs

☐ Coriander

MENU: WEEK 1

	Breakfast	Lunch	Dinner
Saturday	Banana and cardamom bread	Chicken gado-gado	'Turkey' turkey burgers
Sunday	Spanikopita (feta and spinach breakfast pastries)	Corn chowder soup	Pork and preserved lemon tagine with roasted kale
Monday	Strawberries, cream cheese and cocoa nibs on toast	Bruschetta with mozzarella	Artichoke, garlic and cream cheese pizzas
Tuesday	One-pan bacon and eggs	Nutty mango, avocado and quinoa salad	'Steak'wiches
Wednesday	Nutty granola	Broad bean, artichoke and feta salad	Herby salmon en croute
Thursday	Plum and pistachio chia pudding	Smoked mackerel and new potato salad	Shepherd-less pie
Friday	Nutty 'carrot cake' porridge	Spiced carrot and lentil salad with halloumi and peanut dressing	Crispy fish finger sandwiches with homemade tartare sauce

MENU: WEEK 2

	Breakfast	Lunch	Dinner
Saturday	Blackberry and apple breakfast 'crumble'	Avgolemono soup	Chicken tamarind curry
Sunday	Rye bread with avocado, bacon and cherry tomatoes	Warm lentil and halloumi salad with a zingy preserved lemon dressing	Wholewheat pasta with roast pork meatballs and gremolata
Monday	Pomegranate and tahini chia pudding	Roast vegetable salad with kale and hazelnut pesto	Quinoa bowl with sticky aubergines, hummus and feta
Tuesday	Kale and Parmesan scrambled eggs	Bulgur wheat, feta and olive salad with hummus	Prawn and chorizo paella
Wednesday	Caramelised banana and cocoa nib porridge	Aubergine, sweetcorn and avocado wraps	Salmon tacos
Thursday	Healthy beans on toast	Nutty kale and chorizo salad with sriracha	Sweet potato burgers with a melting goat's cheese centre
Friday	Raspberry, almond and mint chia pudding	Soft cheese and roasted cherry tomato tartine	Chicken, sweet potato and tarragon traybake

MENU: WEEK 3

	Breakfast	Lunch	Dinner
Saturday	Healthy breakfast muffins	Spanish omelette	Harissa-baked chicken with flatbreads and salad
Sunday	Spicy baked eggs with chorizo and halloumi	Spicy shredded Vietnamese chicken salad	Beef massaman curry
Monday	Apple and sultana bircher muesli	Chicken, feta and lettuce pitta pockets	Chicken laksa
Tuesday	Egg in a cup	Avocado, mango and cucumber salad	Beef and lentil cottage pie with roasted broccoli
Wednesday	Mango and coconut bircher muesli	Roasted broccoli and goat's cheese tartine	Ginger and soy steamed sea bass
Thursday	Egg-in-a-hole with cherry tomato salsa	Beetroot and feta wrap	Sweet potato dhal with toasted coconut flakes
Friday	Creamy porridge with berry jam	Cucumber, cream cheese and dill bagels	Grilled tuna steaks with a cherry tomato salsa

MENU: WEEK 4

	Breakfast	Lunch	Dinner
Saturday	Buttermilk rusks with cranberries and pistachios	Tom yum soup	Pesto and chicken crumble with green salad
Sunday	Green mushroom and ricotta crêpes	One-pot roast chicken	Sundried tomato and mozzarella tart with rocket and walnut pesto
Monday	Apricot, blueberry and hazelnut chia pudding	Peach, mozzarella and Parma ham salad	Harissa-marinated lamb kebabs with Greek salad
Tuesday	Menemen	Pesto chickpea salad with cherry tomatoes	Chicken skewers with rainbow slaw and warm pittas
Wednesday	Porridge with rhubarb and ginger	Artichoke, broad bean and feta salad	Smoked mackerel kedgeree
Thursday	Spicy scrambled eggs	Roast vegetable and goat's cheese frittata	Asparagus and lemon pearl barley risotto
Friday	Carrot and sultana drop scones	Ricotta, pea and asparagus tartine	Hake with hasselback potatoes and braised veggies

MENU: WEEK 5

	Breakfast	Lunch	Dinner
Saturday	Crumpet French toast with whipped ricotta and berries	Smoked chicken quesadilla	Aubergine Parmigiana
Sunday	Breakfast burritos	Rainbow vegetable tart	Mushroom, kale and Cheddar savoury oatmeal